TU YOUYOU'S JOURNEY IN THE SEARCH FOR ARTEMISININ

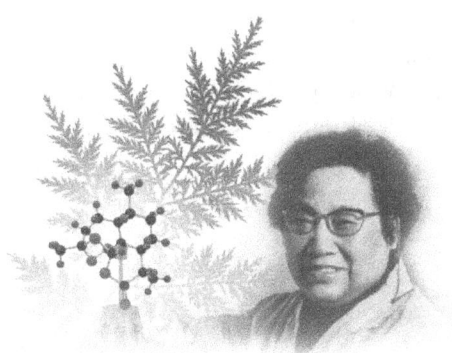

TU YOUYOU'S JOURNEY IN THE SEARCH FOR ARTEMISININ

Wenhu Zhang
Chemical Industry Press, China

Yiran Shao
Chemical Industry Press, China

Dan Li
Beijing Television Station, China

Manyuan Wang
Capital Medical University, China

Translated by: Junxian Yu
Capital Medical University, China

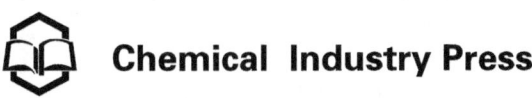

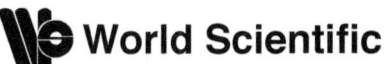

NEW JERSEY · LONDON · SINGAPORE · BEIJING · SHANGHAI · HONG KONG · TAIPEI · CHENNAI · TOKYO

Published by

World Scientific Publishing Co. Pte. Ltd.
5 Toh Tuck Link, Singapore 596224
USA office: 27 Warren Street, Suite 401-402, Hackensack, NJ 07601
UK office: 57 Shelton Street, Covent Garden, London WC2H 9HE

and

Chemical Industry Press
No. 13, Qingnianhu South Street
Dongcheng District, Beijing 100011
P. R. China

Library of Congress Cataloging-in-Publication Data
Names: Hu, Zhiqiang, 1964–   author.
Title: Tu Youyou's journey in the search for artemisinin / by Zhiqiang Hu,
    Dan Li, Manyuan Wang, Lan Yang, Yansong Li, Yiran Shao, Wenhu Zhang.
Description: New Jersey : World Scientific, 2017.
Identifiers: LCCN 2017001762| ISBN 9789813207639 (hardcover : alk. paper) |
    ISBN 9789813207646 (pbk. : alk. paper)
Subjects: | MESH: Tu, Youyou, 1930- | Artemisinins--history | Antimalarials--history |
    Drug Discovery--history | Malaria--history | Nobel Prize | History, 20th Century |
    History, 21st Century | China | Biography
Classification: LCC RS420 | NLM QV 256 | DDC 615.1/9--dc23
LC record available at https://lccn.loc.gov/2017001762

British Library Cataloguing-in-Publication Data
A catalogue record for this book is available from the British Library.

B&R Book Program

Copyright © 2018 by World Scientific Publishing Co. Pte. Ltd. and Chemical Industry Press

All rights reserved. This book, or parts thereof, may not be reproduced in any form or by any means, electronic or mechanical, including photocopying, recording or any information storage and retrieval system now known or to be invented, without written permission from the publisher.

For photocopying of material in this volume, please pay a copying fee through the Copyright Clearance Center, Inc., 222 Rosewood Drive, Danvers, MA 01923, USA. In this case permission to photocopy is not required from the publisher.

The First Chinese Female Nobel Laureate's Search for Artemisinin

*An inspirational story of a female scientist.
A less known and difficult history of malaria in China.
Facing divergent controversies, she pressed on,
"I will just learn more."
Thereafter she kept silent.*

Preface

Zhang Wenhu

This book tells the discovery story of the legendary drug — artemisinin. It is the story of Tu Youyou, who, as we know, shared the 2015 Nobel Prize in Physiology/Medicine with William Campbell and Satoshi Omura, for discovering artemisinin, a drug against malaria.

Ms. Tu had been unwilling to tell her own story for a long time. The day after the announcement of her Nobel Prize win, she finally told journalists to read her book, *Artemisia Annua and Artemisinin-Based Drugs*, which I had edited and Chemical Industry Press had published. I had been fortunate enough to work with Ms. Tu and through the process, came to know the winding twists and turns in her complex and vivid story.

The period of history covered in this book spans a particular era and was generated from a miserable war; it was closely related to the secret "Project 523", and involved various institutions and individuals in China. The story reads like a stage drama, with vibrant stage background, a melodious accompaniment chorus, and various types of roles, all of which push the development of the story. Nevertheless, we know that the soul of every drama is the life of the protagonist, and what happens to whom is the plotline. This drama is about the scientific discovery of a Chinese scientist.

A great discovery is always an unpredictable result of many active and passive conditions. It is inseparable from the intelligence and wisdom, as well as tough character of the discoverer; and it very often requires a bit of luck. Especially in major scientific discoveries, scientists may rack their brains, but inspiration may only be gained under accidental circumstances. Such discoveries may seem to be the inconceivable strokes of genius, but in fact, they are a leap of creative thinking by the scientists. As mentioned in the book, the therapy of treating malaria with artemisia annua has a history of over thousands of years in China, and numerous scientists have tried to find effective methods for treating malaria, but why was the key breakthrough made by Tu Youyou? Was it purely a coincidental discovery? Or did it stem from basic logic?

The mission of scientists is to discover the natural mysteries, but their discovery process is also a mystery. It is the task of epistemology to solve this mystery. Over two thousand years, philosophers have undertaken various studies on knowledge acquisition of human beings, and come up with many original ideas and incisive comments.

John Locke advocated empiricism, referring to the theory "knowledge derives from experience"; Plato and Kant advocated rationalism, referring to the theory "knowledge is priori"; and Hume advocated skepticism, referring to the theory of "questioning human beings' inductive ability of promoting the empirical observation to universal rules". In the process of stating their philosophical viewpoints, these philosophers expressed their excellent deductive competence and rational brilliance, as well as their understanding of human knowledge and humanity, all of which are worthy of our attention.

Nevertheless, empiricism and rationalism are unable to fully solve the mystery of scientific discovery. From empiricism, one would pay attention to the ancient records and empirical formulas for treating malaria with artemisia annua, and the hundreds of experiments of "Project 523", whilst neglecting the key discoverer and her key achievements. From rationalism, one would focus on the abstract reasoning of Ms. Tu, thus resulting in an over-emphasis on the unusual rational intuitive ability of scientists. However, after reading this book, it is clear that empiricism and rationalism cannot provide a complete and fully accurate picture to explain the discovery of artemisinin: although many scientists were aware of the ancient records about artemisia annua and its application by folk doctors, and many others conducted experiments on pepper, antifebrile dichroa and even tried acupuncture, only Tu Youyou continued the research on artemisia annua, and finally discovered artemisinin.

Therefore, I would like to introduce the opinion of Karl Popper, one of the greatest philosophers of science of the 20th century, on scientific discovery. In *The Logic of Scientific Discovery*, Popper proposed an opinion differing from empiricism and rationalism, and then formulated his theory of falsificationism. He believed scientific discovery was neither promoted to laws and theories through the inductive method after collecting large numbers of observations or through empirical materials as stated by empiricism, nor inferred through the inductive method on the basis of a priori truths as stated by rationalism; instead, it was a process following a model of "conjectures and refutations".

As far as Popper was concerned, scientific research did not derive from observation or some a priori truths, but from questions. Scientific questions arise from incomplete theoretical or practical knowledge. In order to answer these questions, scientists propose hypotheses through speculation. Of course, not all hypotheses are scientific ones, in principle, only the ones that can be proven false (falsification) by experience are scientific hypotheses. Next, the scientists verify the hypotheses, to find out whether they are false. If they are indeed proven to be false, the scientists would propose new hypotheses. Through constant conjectures and refutations, scientists promote the advancement of science.

With the help of Popper's model of "conjectures and refutations", we may better understand the keys to the discovery of artemisinin. Social demand at the time underscored to Chinese scientists the need to search for an effective cure. Ms. Tu's unique role was in proposing and following up on the conjecture that was proven to be effective later. At the time, Project 523 had many investigative directions, Ms. Tu was responsible for screening Chinese medical herbs; in consideration of her responsibility for testing the selected herbs and observing the final results, she was required to treat each kind of medicinal herbs objectively, without bias. Therefore, she initially wrote off artemisia annua like pepper, because the effect of their initial extracts was less than satisfactory. Given this circumstance and the existence of thousands of Chinese medicinal herbs, the discovery of artemisinin could just as well have not happened. Nevertheless, Ms. Tu started reflecting at a certain stage during her research, the motivation of her reflection might have come from a sense of failure, responsibility or duty toward her organization. But at that moment, Ms. Tu unconsciously arrived at the point of proposing a "hypothesis", a situation familiar to all scientists. Perhaps it was inspiration, perhaps intuition, just a few words in a historical record gave her the idea for the hypothesis: "the low temperature extraction method may extract the active substances from artemisia annua"; it was also at that moment that she made a great leap in creative thinking.

Her unique role in the discovery of artemisinin was also reflected in her trying of every means to verify this hypothesis; the verifying process was a little different from that advocated by empiricism. The verification in this case was designed to be more comprehensive, intricate and partial, to be convenient for observation, rejection and acceptance. This is the reason why there were so many processes for verifying artemisia annua. For example, in designing an experiment for distinguishing the roots, stems and leaves of artemisia annua, the harvest time also had to be considered. In addition to ether, more solvents with low boiling points were also used; the negative answers contrary to the expectation became the driving force of research, instead of being sources of discouragement for the scientists.

The discovery of artemisinin has experienced several cycles from conjecture to hypotheses verification, an undulating and complex process requiring various forces to jointly promote its development. Organizations or institutions played an important supportive role, such as in promoting reflection; the ancient and modern scientific resources or resources of traditional Chinese medicine also aided in scientific discovery, such as in promoting hypotheses formation; the research teams also had their part to play, such as in the inspection and trial & error process. But the entire process of making an original discovery cannot be separated from the directive force that comes from the scientist, because the formulation and verification of hypotheses do not have any mechanical process, but have an obvious relationship with the intellectual capacity and determination of a scientist. It is often said that the earth will still rotate without anyone. But it is hard to imagine the history of science without Newton, Darwin, and Einstein. In my opinion, the discovery of artemisinin is closely related to the strong will, timely reflection, rational hypotheses, and detailed examination of Ms. Tu, factors that are strongly associated with scientists as individuals.

After winning the Nobel Prize, Ms. Tu expressed that the successful discovery of artemisinin was the result of collective research and that it was a collective honor to Chinese scientists. I believe this is a pertinent yet modest statement. In the discovery process of artemisinin, the "collective research" organized by the 523 Office, the "large-scale cooperation" between various institutions, and unified efforts of the research teams made great contributions, thus they certainly deserve social praise and reward. However, such achievements are different in nature from the unique and original contribution of Ms. Tu. In our society, a number of people typically downplay and disregard the creative capacities of scientists, which is why I emphasize her originality, for originality is the essential core of scientific research.

This book focuses on the main character who contributed to the discovery of artemisinin and the exploration process of scientific discovery; it tries to reveal the basic logic and essential characteristics of scientific discovery, to lead young readers to the answer of the question "Why was it Tu Youyou who discovered artemisinin?", thereby enabling them to more profoundly understand the original features of scientific research. This experimental approach is also what makes it stand out from other similar publications. The most remarkable feature of Ms. Tu is her practice of preserving all the collected materials and her habit of timely record keeping, which has allowed for the discovery history of artemisinin to be completely and clearly presented. In narrating this process, the writers have tried their best to restore the details of the relevant incidents and activities. But some details are not easily comprehensible, such as psychological activities; therefore, they are not included in the book given space constraints. Irrelevant or unimportant details have also been omitted. In order to ensure the coherence of the story, consultation of the appropriate literature was beneficial. As aside from the purpose of increasing knowledge, the more important goal of popular science is to instruct and inspire.

Zhang Wenhu
March 2016

Contents

Preface vii

Beginning from the Nobel Prize 1
Setting Ambition at a Young Age 5
Studying at Peking University 11
Wholeheartedly Moving Forward 17
Encountering "Project 523" 25
Horrible Malaria 31
History of the Antimalarial Fight 35
War and Malaria 43
The Launch of Antimalarial Research 47
Inspiration and Success 53
Specimen 191 57
Experiments on Laboratory Rats 61
Personally Testing Efficacy 65

Antimalarial Symphony	71
From Crystal to Drug	75
Unique Artemisinin	81
Rectification of the Name of *Artemisia annua* L.	87
Each Showing Its Special Prowess	91
Introduction into Africa	101
Looking for the Discoverer	107
Winning the Nobel Prize	111
Epilogue	115

Beginning from the Nobel Prize

This is not only an honor for me, but also the recognition of and motivation for all scientists in China.

Getting Informed about Winning the Nobel Prize

On October 5, 2015, it was a slightly cool autumn evening. "At 5:30 p.m. (Beijing Time), the 2015 Nobel Prize in Physiology/Medicine was announced, and Tu Youyou, a famous Chinese scientist, was awarded the Prize in Medicine for discovering artemisinin, a new drug against malaria, which enabled the first Chinese citizen to win a Nobel Prize in Medicine…"

TV cameras were zooming in, giving a close-up shot of Tu's withered facial features; the curly grey hair, steady gaze, as well as deep forehead wrinkles, expressed her fortitude. Tu had been conducting research on artemisinin through combining Chinese traditional medicine and new drugs over several decades, leading to the discovery of artemisinin, a new drug with good curative effect against malaria, which has saved millions of lives.

Award Ceremony

At about 11:30 p.m. (Beijing Time) on December 10, 2015, the 2015 Nobel Prize Award Ceremony was held at the Stockholm Concert Hall in Sweden. Ten laureates of the 2015 Nobel Prize in Literature, Physics, Chemistry, Physiology/Medicine, and Economic Sciences attended the award ceremony from all over the world; the eldest among them was Chinese scientist Tu Youyou.

At the moment of accepting the prize, Tu Youyou, dressed in a purple suit, stepped up to the podium and received the medal and certificate of Nobel Prize from Carl XVI Gustaf, King of Sweden. It was a historic moment for the world and especially for China; it was the first time that a Chinese scientist was receiving the Nobel Prize in Science.

A Gift from Traditional Chinese Medicine to the World

On the afternoon of December 7, Tu Youyou made an excellent speech entitled *Artemisinin — A Gift from Traditional Chinese Medicine to the World* at the Karolinska Institute in Sweden. During her 26-minute-long speech, Jan Andersson, host of the Nobel Prize Keynote Speech and Professor of Lemology at Karolinska Institute, got down unhesitatingly on one knee to hold the microphone for the 85-year-old Tu Youyou:

> This is not only an honor for me, but also the recognition of and motivation for all scientists in China.
>
> [...]
>
> I would like to express my sincere gratitude again to my fellow colleagues of Project 523 at the Academy of Traditional Chinese Medicine, for their active devotion and outstanding contributions to the discovery and subsequent applications of artemisinin. I would like to thank the units of Project 523, including the Shandong Provincial Institute of Chinese Medicine, Yunnan Provincial Institute of Materia Medica, Institute of Biophysics of the Chinese Academy of Sciences, Shanghai Institute of Organic Chemistry of the Chinese Academy of Sciences, the Guangzhou University of Chinese Medicine, and the Academy of Military Medical Sciences for their full cooperation; I would also like to

sincerely congratulate all colleagues on their invaluable achievements and heartfelt service toward malaria patients. I would like to express my sincere respect for the continuous efforts of the National 523 Office in organizing antimalarial projects. Without this selfless and cooperative spirit, we would not be able to present artemisinin to the world in such a short term.

"Chinese traditional medicine is a great treasure for all medical workers to learn and explore, we should improve it to a higher level." Artemisinin is an effective drug discovered from this treasure. Through the research involved in the discovery of artemisinin, we learnt strengths in both Chinese and Western medicines. If these strengths can be fully integrated, there would be even greater potential and better prospects [for health]. Nature provides us with a large number of plant resources, from which medical researchers can develop novel medicines. Traditional Chinese medicine, since "Shen Nong Tastes Hundreds of Herbs", has accumulated substantial clinical experience in its development over thousands of years, and has also sorted and summarized the medicinal values of natural resources. Through inheriting, developing, exploring and improving, we can discover new medicines beneficial to mankind.

Setting Ambition at a Young Age

As an old Chinese saying goes, "Misfortune may be an actual blessing". In her youth, Tu Youyou narrowly escaped death from pulmonary tuberculosis and her experience led her to become greatly interested in medicine; this seed of passion, deeply embedded in her heart, became the source of her undying faith and strength. Thereafter, Tu Youyou focused single-mindedly on how to absorb more knowledge about medicine.

A Severe Disease

In 1946, 16-year-old Tu Youyou was compelled to interrupt her education due to infection with pulmonary tuberculosis, a kind of chronic infectious disease, which given the level of medical treatment at that time, was almost impossible to be cured.

Despite the tense political situation and difficult family circumstances, her parents did not give up and spared no efforts to cure her. She still remembers what she asked while watching the vapor rising from the cup offered by her mother Yao Zhongqian, "Mom, am I going to die?"

"Don't talk nonsense, you will get well, and there are numerous things for you to do!"

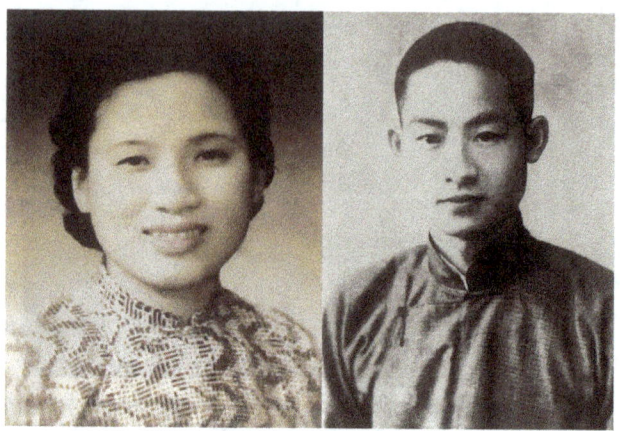

Tu Youyou's parents: Yao Zhongqian and Tu Liangui.

"I will get well and be healthy!" she resolved there and then.

Thanks to her strong will to survive and her parents' meticulous care, she miraculously recovered after more than two years of treatment with Chinese medicine.

On the Origins of Tu Youyou's Name

The Tu family lived at No. 508, Kaiming Street, Ningbo City, Zhejiang Province, China. On December 30, 1930, they finally welcomed a daughter, after three sons.

Father Tu named his little daughter Youyou, following a tradition of "naming a girl after *The Book of Songs*, and a boy after *The Songs of Chu*". Her cute name was from *The Book of Songs ·Xiao Ya · Lu Ming*, which, also quoted by Cao Cao in his well known *Duangexing*, refers to "deer call". As far as naming for a girl is concerned, "deer call" can be said to symbolize a lively, bold, lovely and optimistic character. However, beyond Tu Liangui's expectation, his daughter not only possessed the traits he desired, she also became a great scientist. In fact, the lyrics from *The Book of Songs* "With pleased sounds the deer call to one another, eating *Artemisia annua* of the fields, I have here admirable guests, whose virtuous fame is grandly brilliant" seem to predict the connection between artemisinin and Tu Youyou more than two thousand years later.

Turbulence and Disease

Tu Youyou spent her childhood in an age of turbulence. China suffered from the wars and people lived in abject poverty. Ningbo, due to its coastal location, was naturally a strategic area that Japan wanted to occupy. When the city eventually fell into Japanese hands, all its citizens, including the Tu family, could no longer live ordinary lives. Thereafter, the family of six, which had not been wealthy to begin with, were forced into an impoverished wartime existence.

In 1941, Tu Youyou, together with her parents, moved to her maternal grandparents' house, No. 26, Kaiming Street, for they could no longer live in their original house. She stayed there in the house built by her grandpa Yao Yongbai until 1951 when she entered university.

Regardless of the tense political situation and their difficult family circumstances, Tu's parents, disregarding the feudal saying that "Innocence is a virtue for women", believed in the importance of schooling, and they sent Tu Youyou to school when she was five to begin her education. After kindergarten, she entered Ningbo Private Chongde Lower Primary School at six; five years later, she was sent to Ningbo Private Maoxi Higher Primary School. At age 13, she entered Ningbo Private Qizhen Middle School, and then went on to study at Ningbo Private Yongjiang Middle School for Girls at age 15. However, as mentioned, her schooling was interrupted by pulmonary tuberculosis when she was 16, causing much anxiety to her family.

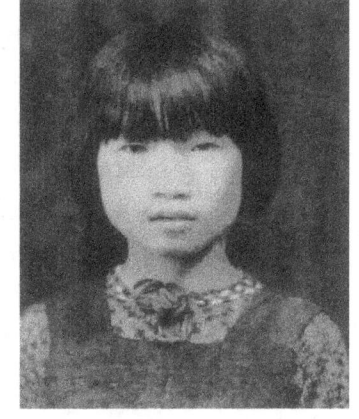

Tu Youyou as a child.

The Beginning of a Dream

After her recovery, Tu Youyou enrolled in Ningbo Private Xiaoshi Senior High School in February 1948.

Xiaoshi High School, founded by physicists He Yujie, Ye Bingliang, Chen Xunzheng and Qian Baohang with the support of a local patron Li Jingdi in February 1912, was a well-known school at that time. With its mission of "implementing education with private strength, to make a way for rule of the people", it educated a large number of students who were highly regarded. By 1917, it had signed agreements with Fudan University and St. John's University, the two elite universities in Shanghai. These agreements allowed graduates from Xiaoshi High School to be enrolled into either university without taking further examinations.

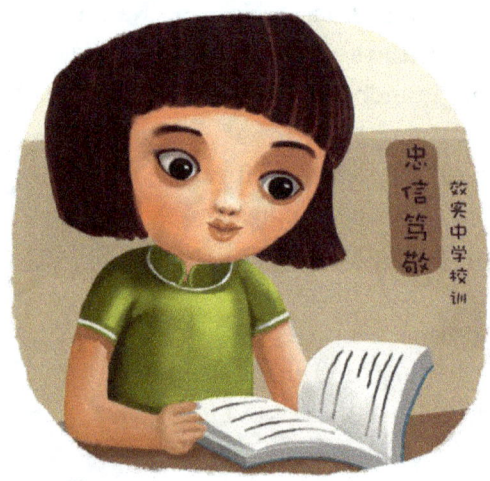

Motto of Xiaoshi High School: Be Faithful, Honest, Earnest and Reverent (drawn by Zhang Linhao).

As an old Chinese saying goes, "Misfortune may be an actual blessing". In her youth, Tu Youyou narrowly escaped death from pulmonary tuberculosis and her experience led her to become greatly interested in medicine; this seed of passion, deeply embedded in her heart, became the source of her undying faith and strength.

Thereafter, Tu Youyou focused single-mindedly on how to absorb more knowledge about medicine.

In the eyes of her classmates, she was simple and quiet; compared to some other female classmates who gained fame in school for their participation in drama performances, she was unobtrusive, often observed studying silently and tenaciously in a corner of the classroom.

As recalled by Chen Xiaozhong, her high school classmate and professor of Tsinghua University, Tu Youyou, being plain and simply dressed, always studied hard in silence, and went home directly after school, in a word, she was a simple girl. At that time, she certainly would not have imagined that Li Tingzhao, her male classmate in high school, would become her husband.

At school, Tu Youyou's results were not the highest, though they hovered around the middle–upper level in the class. Based on the information preserved in the Ningbo Archives, the average scores of Tu Youyou, student ID No. A342, in Chinese, Mathematics, Biology and Chemistry were respectively 71.25, 71.5, 80.5 and 67.5; with the average score of Biology being the highest.

Some may consider such results too mediocre for a Nobel Prize winner. Nevertheless, despite being rather ordinary during her school days, Tu Youyou clearly demonstrated her great enthusiasm and persistence for knowledge, the exact characteristics shared by numerous scientists.

In March 1950, Tu Youyou transferred to Ningbo High School. Driven by the pursuit of a dream, her thirst for knowledge, and deep respect for medical science, Tu Youyou completed her high school life. At that time, no one expected that this unassuming girl would eventually achieve academic results good enough for her to be admitted to Peking University; no one could guess that she would select the relatively unpopular and newly established College of Medicine; and certainly no one could imagine that she would win the remarkable Nobel Prize 55 years later.

Today, the house of her childhood — The Yao's House — has been renamed as "Tu Youyou's Former Residence"; her works have been widely circulated, and her pictures have flooded media channels. All of this have just one source of origin: that pure but invaluable seed of dream that she buried in her heart during childhood.

Studying at Peking University

―――❈―――

While her schoolmates were basking in varsity life, Tu Youyou was always to be found in the classroom, attentively acquiring knowledge. In Tu's world, the campus was not a place for her to waste her youth, and in fact, "pharmacognosy" was her entire world. For this young girl on the road of realizing a dream, every step she took was steadfast and firm.

Entering Peking University

In the summer of 1951, with the founding of New China, many things were waiting to be done and professionals were required in all fields. High school graduates at that time were spoilt for choice, they could major in popular fields such as economic management and motor science. Unexpectedly, Tu Youyou, coming from a family background with no medical tradition or experience, selected medicine in her application for university.

In late summer, Tu Youyou received her letter of admission from Peking University's College of Medicine; she became one of the first batch of female college students in China. We can only imagine how joyful and proud the 21-year-old girl was.

Peking University, at that time, had just completed the lengthy and complex readjustment of colleges and departments and had moved to the location of the former Yenching University. Social scientists gathered at Peking University like soldiers answering to the call of assembly. From then on, Peking University became one of the "Two Top-Ranking Academic Institutions" in China, even to this day.

Peking University's College of Medicine was affiliated with Peking University Medical School, which was located near The North Church in Xicheng District, the location of Peking University's School of Stomatology's Primary Clinic today.

Selecting Pharmacognosy

After enrollment, Tu Youyou was assigned to Medicine Class 8 with over seventy classmates; they studied together in the first three years, and then chose their specializations in the fourth year. There were three majors at that time: medicinal examination, medicinal chemistry and pharmacognosy. Tu Youyou, with another 11 classmates, selected pharmacognosy, while the most popular choice was medicinal chemistry.

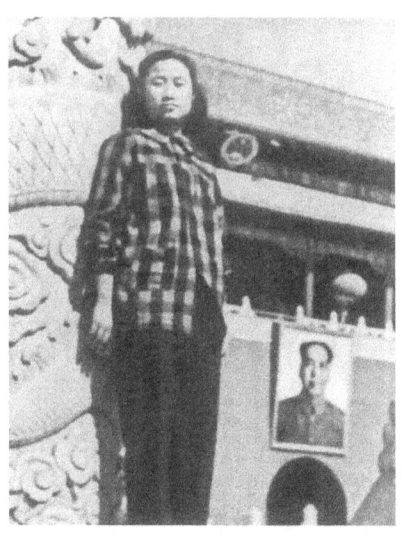

Tu Youyou at Tiananmen Square during her varsity days in Peking University.

Pharmacognosy, in brief, is the specialty of classifying and identifying various natural medicines, which means that students specializing in this field would mainly carry out research on medicines after graduation; Tu's selection conformed to her quiet personality.

Pharmacognosy was just unfolding at that time. All of what she saw was new to her: the laboratory equipment, the aged buildings housing more modern facilities... the reagent constantly changing colors in test tubes, the active cells under the microscope, and microorganisms moving in petri dishes; everything was exciting to her. On this campus pervaded with an atmosphere of strong academic tradition, Tu Youyou embarked on the most important learning journey of her life.

At Peking University, Tu Youyou, like in high school, remained humble and diligent; it seemed like she was born to engage in academic research. The quiet girl continued to prefer solitude as in her youth. It was rare to find her at places of entertainment, instead she would usually be inhabiting a corner of the library, reading and thinking. While her schoolmates were basking in varsity life, Tu Youyou was always to be found in the classroom, attentively acquiring knowledge. In Tu's world, the campus was not a place for her to waste her youth, and in fact, "pharmacognosy" was her entire world. For this young girl on the road of realizing a dream, every step she took was steadfast and firm.

The Legendary Professor Lou Zhicen

The legendary Professor Lou Zhicen, was the one who established the pharmacognosy specialty in Peking University. His own learning experience was truly an inspirational story of passion that impelled many pharmacognosy majors to courageously move forward on this road.

Lou Zhicen, born in Anji County, Zhejiang Province on January 28, 1920, went to study at the School of Pharmacy, University of London in September 1945 when he was 25 years old. He achieved excellent results and obtained his Bachelor's degree two years later. However, his scholarship from the British Council was to expire in the summer of the following year, and he was faced with the prospect of having to prematurely discontinue his studies.

Fortunately, it was not long afterwards that his benefactor appeared. With his outstanding performance and enthusiasm in research work, he caught the attention of J. W. Fairbairn, Professor of Pharmacognosy at the University of London. The university had never hired any non-British research assistant before, but through the tireless lobbying efforts of Fairbairn, a new precedent was set and Lou Zhicen was hired as a Research Assistant of Pharmacognosy at the University of London, whilst simultaneously working toward his Doctoral degree. Thus, it was thanks to the help of J. W. Fairbairn that Lou Zhicen could continue living and studying at the university.

With such encouragement, Lou Zhicen poured his heart into research and study. Finally, in 1950, he completed his doctoral thesis, in addition to six research papers. More importantly, under the encouragement and guidance of Professor J. W. Fairbairn, he also completed a whole series of research work. During that period, he established a new bioassay method for botanical laxatives, which was published in 1949 in an academic journal specializing in the field. His method opened up intense discussion among scholars from various countries; subsequently these scholars began to use this method widely for their own research. This became known as the famous "Lou's Method" in the field of pharmacognosy; it can effectively and accurately measure and separate active ingredients in medicinal materials with an advanced and efficient technology, thus improving the stability and accuracy of measurement.

The British academia and industry realized the talent of Lou Zhicen, and Professor J. W. Fairbairn, not wanting to lose such a talent, entreated Lou to remain in Britain to do more research work with him. A few days later, Lou also received an invitation from Evans Pharmaceutical Factory with an irresistible annual salary. Regardless, despite the two very attractive offers, Lou Zhicen, as other patriotic scientists before him, chose to return home to China. In January 1951, enheartened by his deep loyalty to his country, he boarded a passenger ship sailing to Hong Kong.

After a long trip, Lou Zhicen finally arrived in Shanghai from Hong Kong. Sun Zongpeng, Director of the College of Medicine, Faculty of Science at Zhejiang University wasted no time in sending Lou an invitation to further his research at the university. Sun Zongpeng, already an admirer of Lou's capabilities, spoke with conviction about the situation of New China and the academic circle to be constructed. After listening to Sun, Lou Zhicen did not say anything but merely nodded. And so, he came to be appointed Associate Professor at the College of Medicine in Zhejiang University, to temporarily teach pharmacy to the graduating students. That autumn, Lou Zhicen, after his brief stint at Zhejiang University, moved to the College of Medicine, Beijing Medical College (now the Peking University Health Science Center), and he established the Pharmacognosy Teaching and Research Office.

Years later, Lou Zhicen became a pharmacognosy scientist and pharmaceutical educator, and he was selected as one of the first batch of academicians at the Chinese Academy of Engineering (CAE) Medical and Health Engineering Department, as well as the academic leader of the national key discipline of pharmacognosy. In China, he is undoubtedly one of the "founders" of pharmacognosy.

Mentor Lin Qishou

Another important course — phytochemistry — was established by Lin Qishou who returned to China after studying in the United States. Lin Qishou studied pharmacology at the College of Medicine, University of Maryland in June 1949, and as a researcher, he mainly engaged in synthesis research on narcotics. He returned to China in March 1950, and served as Associate Professor in the College of Medicine at Peking University's Health Science Center.

In Tu Youyou's memory, Lin always explained the interesting knowledge about medicinal chemistry and phytochemistry in simple and humorous language, which benefited all students a lot. Tu Youyou still remembers his operation of segregating herb ingredients with chromatography.

> *Of all the courses in the major, pharmacognosy and phytochemistry were most useful for her future work in drug research; they provided her with the right mentality, direction and methods in the process of her study and discovery of artemisinin. Years later, Tu Youyou, in retrospect, said that majoring in pharmacognosy had indeed been a very important choice that she had made.*

Wholeheartedly Moving Forward

Many years later, Li Jun, the younger daughter of Tu Youyou, expressed her feelings and the confusion that beset her in an interview, "They were strangers to me at that time, and mom and dad had no special meanings to me. I just could not understand how they could abandon their family and even children for scientific research." From Tu Youyou's perspective, "When there was any conflict between life and career, we always put career first, and first got the work done."

Beginning of Work

In 1955, Tu Youyou, after completing her undergraduate studies, was assigned to work in the Institute of Chinese Materia Medica, Academy of Chinese Medical Sciences, Ministry of Health (MOH). Although the environment there was not as picturesque as that of Peking University, it seemed that even the air was pervaded with academic atmosphere. For Tu at that time, this academic research institute was a "dream come true" sanctuary.

It was a critical year for Tu Youyou and also for the Academy of Chinese Medical Sciences. The rapidly developing Academy of Chinese

Medical Sciences was given a timely boost: to support the establishment of the Academy and promote the development of Chinese Materia Medica, the central government had specially selected a number of well-known senior doctors of traditional Chinese medicine, to form a "national team" for Chinese medicinal research. For Tu Youyou, who was just getting started in research on pharmacognosy, this became the first key that opened the door for her to the treasury of traditional Chinese medicine.

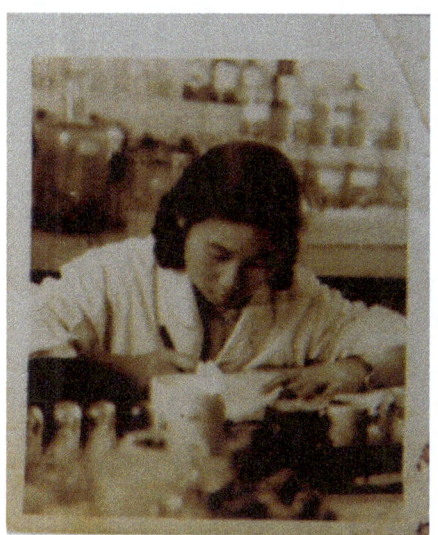
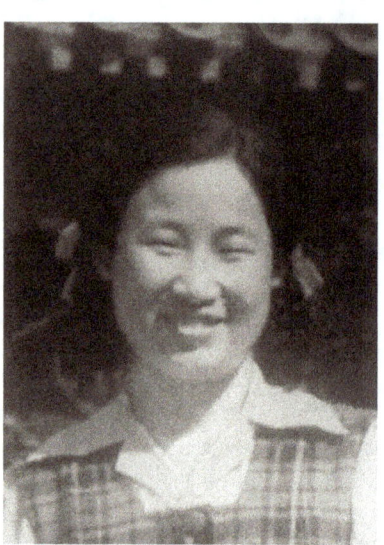

Yu Youyou at her first job.   Tu Youyou in 1957.

In 1956, there was a schistosomiasis outbreak in various parts of China. Inexperienced as she was, Tu Youyou conducted a detailed pharmacognosy research on Chinese lobelia with Professor Lou Zhicen, and gained a fairly good achievement in determining the variety of Chinese lobelia with the best anti-schistosomiasis efficacy.

Before long, inspired by the research on Chinese lobelia, she also completed the pharmacognosy research on starwort root which existed in more complicated varieties. Her research on Chinese lobelia and starwort root, which caused some ripples in the pharmacy circle at that time, were successively included into *Chinese Medicinal Herbal*, a book sorting Chinese medical herbs in combination with modern pharmaceutical achievements. Due to her outstanding performance at work, in 1958, she was lauded as a Socialist Construction Activist by the Ministry of Health.

Participating in "Traditional Chinese Medicine Training Workshops for Western Medical Doctors"

In 1958, Chairman Mao Zedong pointed out in a speech, "… Chinese medicine and pharmacology is a great treasure-house, and great efforts should be made to explore them and raise them to a higher level." Such an appeal very quickly received favorable responses from the masses. Western medical doctors around the country, in addition to continuing their own work in the Western medical tradition, started participating in various traditional Chinese medicine training workshops for Western medical doctors. Chairman Mao subsequently instructed, "This is a big deal, you must not treat it casually, but actively engage in it." As such, such training was even more widely implemented and became a common practice. Chinese medicine learning from Western medicine also became a trend.

According to historical data, there were over 30 such workshops across China in those years, which trained more than 2,000 Western medical doctors; meanwhile, there were more than 36,000 in-service ones participating in the training. Colleges of medicine and pharmacy also set up various courses on traditional Chinese medicine. Traditional Chinese medical research, after experiencing all kinds of hardships previously, entered into a new era in New China. And Tu Youyou was one of the participants, cautiously and steadfastly approaching the treasure container harboring the top secrets of traditional Chinese medicine.

From 1959 to 1962, Tu Youyou underwent training in the third phase of the "Traditional Chinese Medicine Off-Job Training Workshop for Western Medical Doctors" held by the Academy of Chinese Medical Sciences, Ministry of Health. The programme which lasted for two and a half years laid a solid foundation for her future engagement in Chinese medicine research.

Young Tu Youyou did not just remain in the laboratory, she turned to the outside world to acquire practical knowledge, for "only actual combat gives a soldier experience of the real war". Therefore, in accordance with her own major, she went to medicine companies to learn the technique of identifying and processing of herbs from experienced pharmaceutical workers. These masters with numerous years of experience and the "power of practice" that Tu could not learn from books, wholeheartedly imparted their knowledge to her, and shared with her their interesting stories, as well as various seemingly simple yet miraculous "folk prescriptions". Compared with Western medicine which is based on standards and regularity, there is much that is irregular and non-standard in traditional Chinese medicine. However, sometimes it is exactly the accumulated practical experience and wisdom of Chinese people over several thousand years that saves countless lives. Tu Youyou, like a cactus growing roots in the desert in search of water to absorb, recorded, organised and carefully thought through all of these experiences, then kept the memories close to her heart.

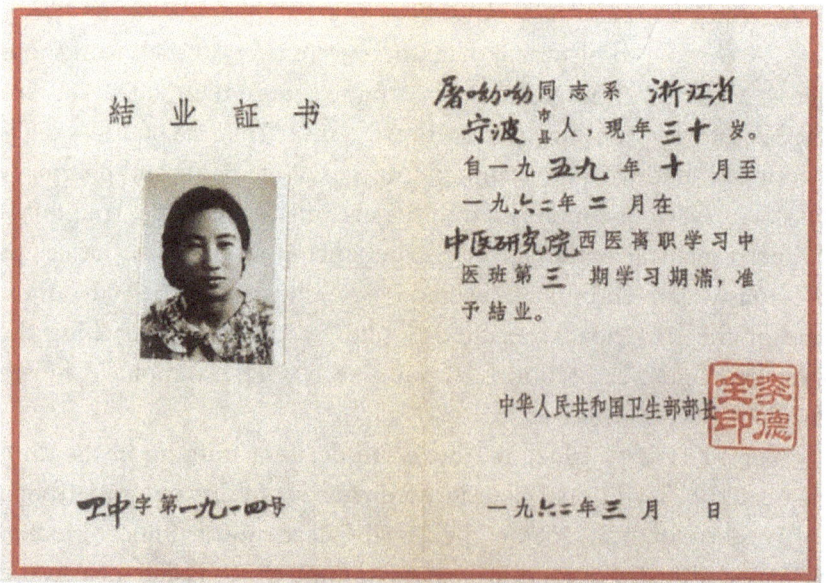

Certificate of completion for Phase III of the "Traditional Chinese Medicine Off-Job Training Workshop for Western Medical Doctors".

In the meantime, she also participated in a roundup of experiences in Chinese herbal medicine processing in Beijing. After returning to theoretical research, she had a deeper understanding of authenticity and quality, as well as the processing technology of medical herbs. Later, Tu Youyou participated in the Chinese herbal medicine processing research organized by the Ministry of Health, and she became one of the main compilers of the book *Chinese Herbal Medicine Processing Experience and Integration*.

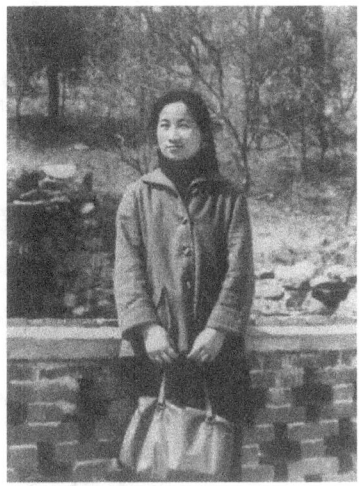

Tu Youyou in 1962

Sacrificing Family for Work

In 1963, Tu Youyou married her high school classmate Li Tingzhao. At that time in China, it was quite rare for a girl to get married only

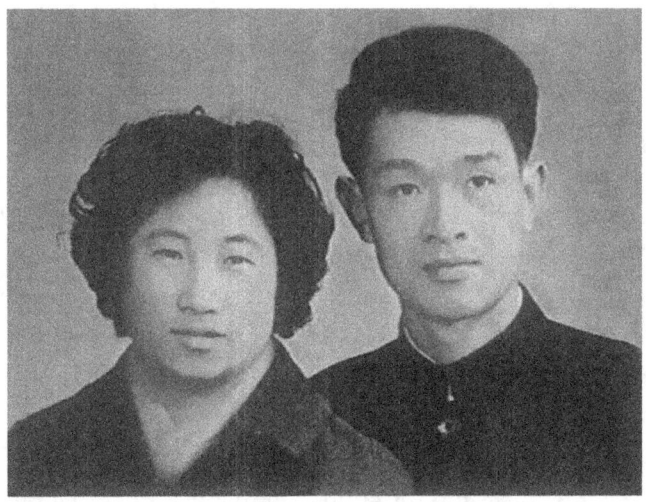

Wedding photo of Tu Youyou and Li Tingzhao.

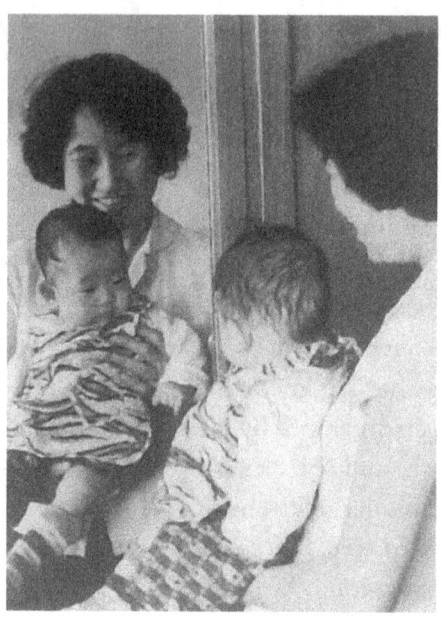

Tu Youyou and her elder daughter Li Min, summer of 1965.

at the age of 33; but Tu Youyou was someone who lived for her work. Being similar to Newton who only concerned himself with physics, Tu was neither good at taking care of herself nor doing housework. Her husband Li Tingzhao, knowing her very well, was understanding and supportive and he took care of all the housework.

In May 1965, their eldest daughter Li Min was born in Beijing. But even before she turned four, she was sent to a full-time childcare facility, as Tu Youyou had to be dispatched to Hainan to conduct some research. Their younger daughter Li Jun, born in September 1968, was sent to Ningbo after birth and looked after by her grandpa Tu Liangui and grandma Yao Zhongqian. The long-term separation created a gap between parents and child; when Tu and her husband were later able to resume taking care of Li Jun, the little girl was unwilling to return to their side.

Many years later, Li Jun, the younger daughter of Tu Youyou, expressed her feelings and the confusion that beset her in an interview, "They were strangers to me at that time, and mom and dad had no

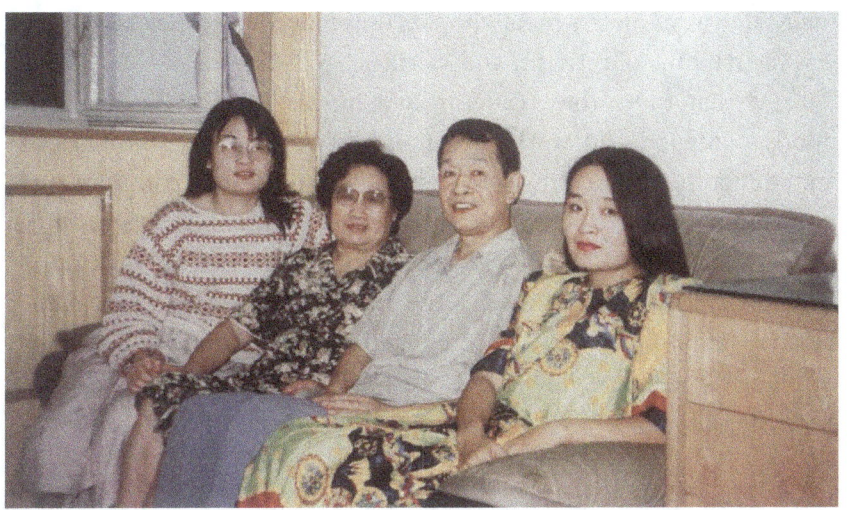

Family photo: Li Jun (left) and Li Min (right), 1996.

special meanings to me. I just could not understand how they could abandon their family and even children for scientific research." From Tu Youyou's perspective: "When there was any conflict between life and career, we always put career first, and first got the work done."

It may be hard for us today to understand why they made the choices they did at that time; however, for people of that generation,

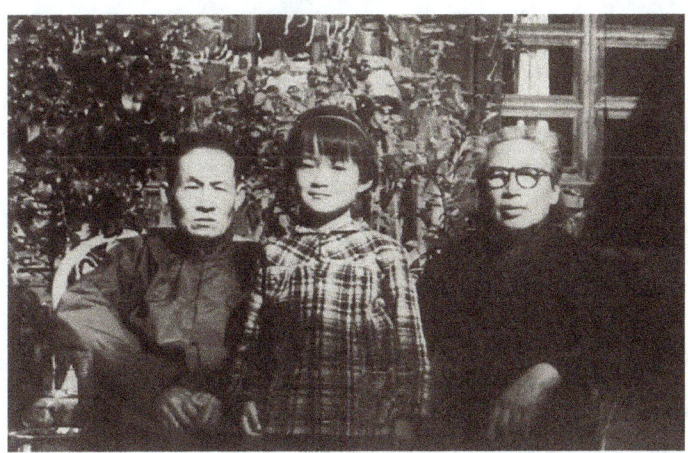

Li Min with her grandpa and grandma, 1974.

their fates were intertwined with the times, and what they believed in was the nation, collectivism and sacrifice.

At that time, the Academy of Chinese Medical Sciences was poorly equipped and working conditions were subpar; the hardship and difficulty in carrying out research under such conditions are unimaginable. But as appraised by Wang Manyuan, a student of Tu, many years later, "Ms. Tu is a particularly persistent, determined and focussed person." Indeed, Tu Youyou has always been such a person, single-mindedly, she completed each collection of specimens, conducted each experiment and wrote each summary analysis, always giving her best effort.

With four years of study at the Peking University Health Science Center, participation in the Traditional Chinese Medicine Training Workshop for Western Medical Doctors, as well as continuous practice at work, the seed of the dream buried deep in Tu's heart had accumulated sufficient energy.

Encountering "Project 523"

From 1965, Tu Youyou began to engage in phytochemistry research, which was also one of the reasons that enabled her to participate in "Project 523". Tu's background was slightly problematic, in the "political" sense: one of her uncles had settled in Hong Kong, and one of her aunts had settled in Taiwan. But in view of her excellent personality, as well as her theoretical research and practical experience in fields of traditional Chinese and Western medicine, Tu Youyou, then a research intern, was selected to lead the antimalarial research team. This marked the start of a brand new page in the history of artemisinin-based antimalarial treatment.

The laboratories in the Academy of Chinese Medical Sciences today are well-equipped and modern in various aspects. As recalled by Tu, when she first began her work there, the laboratory was shabby and the door seemed to isolate two worlds: a secular world outside, and a boring pharmaceutical world inside.

Each time she opens the door, she is engulfed a solemn sense of ritual bringing to mind the time she spent working for Project 523 more than 40 years ago...

Invitation from Project 523

On January 21, 1969, the footsteps of Director Bai Bingqiu and Deputy Director Zhang Jianfang of the Project 523 Office (which had been founded two years ago) and Tian Xin broke the silence of the laboratory at the Academy of Chinese Medical Sciences. They were received by Gao Henian, Deputy Director of the Academy, and Zhang Guozhen, Deputy Director of the Institute of Chinese Materia Medica. After a brief exchange of simple greetings and lighthearted talk, the discussion turned to the serious topic of fighting malaria. Bai Bingqiu said, "Central leaders attach great importance to the research on malaria prevention. We have done much in antimalarial work with traditional Chinese medicine, but the problem has not been resolved. We have little experience and few methods, so we hope you can participate in this effort." The leaders of the Academy pledged to "spare no efforts to undertake the task"; in their minds, they had already silently determined the list of the scientific research team.

Tu Youyou was surprisingly included in this list to undertake the antimalarial mission of China and even the world. From 1965, Tu Youyou began to engage in phytochemistry research, which was also one of the reasons that enabled her to participate in "Project 523". Tu's background was slightly problematic, in the "political" sense: one of her uncles had settled in Hong Kong, and one of her aunts had settled in Taiwan. But in view of her excellent personality, as well as her theoretical research and practical experience in fields of traditional Chinese and Western medicine, Tu Youyou, then a research intern, was selected to lead the antimalarial research team. This marked the start of a brand-new page in the history of artemisinin-based antimalarial treatment.

Origin of "Project 523"

What did the mysterious "Project 523" do? What was Tu Youyou in charge of? The story begins from the Vietnam War.

After World War II, Vietnam, Laos and Cambodia, located in the south of Asia, successively realized independence after expelling the colonists and invaders through armed struggle and uprising. On September 2, 1945, Ho Chi Minh, leader of the Vietnamese Communist Party, declared the foundation of the Democratic Republic of Vietnam in Hanoi. In October 1955, Ngo Dinh Diem founded a new government in Saigon with the support of the United States, creating an antagonistic situation. However, Ngo Dinh Diem's government was contrary to the will of the people; in order to prevent the collapse of Ngo's government, the United States sent a special force named "Green Beret" to South Vietnam in May 1961.

Subsequently, throughout the 1960s, the United States sent more soldiers to Vietnam, further escalating the war.

Both sides suffered a large number of casualties; according to the statistics, over 2 million people died in the war. Falciparum malaria, amidst the hotbed of war, plagued the forces of both sides. As recorded in a relevant report, "For the US army, the non-combat loss rate due to malaria [was] 4–5 times higher than the combat loss rate. In 1965, the annual incidence rate of malaria within the US army in Vietnam reached 50%." As shown by the official data, the US army suffered from around 800,000 deaths due to malaria in the battlefields of Vietnam from 1967 to 1970; in fact, the Director of Preventive Medicine Department, United States Armed Forces Command, once said that the figure far surpassed what was officially announced. Malaria, therefore, was the top military medical problem for US armed forces in Vietnam. Similarly, the forces of North Vietnam also suffered from the malaria-induced losses after entering into South Vietnam.

The spread of malaria in the battlefields of Vietnam had much to do with the local geographical location. The Indochina peninsula, where Vietnam is located, has a tropical hot climate and plentiful rain, in addition to countless mountains and dense forests, mosquitoes may breed regardless of the seasons, thus causing the plague of falciparum malaria throughout the year. Furthermore, the strain in the falciparum malaria plague at that time had a resistance to original antimalarial drugs, which, including chloroquine, pyrimethamine, proguanil and atabrine, could only provide a barely satisfactory therapeutic effect. Therefore, the possession of an efficient, quick, effective and non-resistant antimalarial drug became one of important factors for determining the outcome of war.

To solve this problem, the Americans set up a specialized institution and organized dozens of units to participate in antimalarial research backed by much funding. They repeatedly organized a large number of specialists to carry out medical and epidemiological surveys, as well as experiments on preventive drugs, on the battlefields in Vietnam, and also hired medical experts to serve as medical advisors for malaria prevention and treatment. In addition, they even conducted research on new antimalarial chemical drugs, screening of new antimalarial drugs, and clinical experiments in cooperation with research institutions in Britain, France and Australia, as well as large pharmaceutical companies in Europe.

Vietnam turned to China for help. At the request of the Vietnamese Communist Party, Chairman Mao Zedong and Premier Zhou Enlai instructed the relevant departments to attach importance to the issue of malaria in the tropics and regard malaria treatment and prevention as an urgent combat readiness task of aid for foreign countries.

Significance of "Project 523"

Over time, the development of "Project 523" surpassed the original intention as "aid for Vietnam". In addition to helping China achieve the systematic management of malaria prevention and control, it also promoted the issuance of various malaria prevention and control schemes, and trained many technical personnel in malaria prevention and control. It was as Chairman Mao said, "Solving your problem also means solving of our problem."

In 1964, experts from the Institute of Microbiology and Epidemiology, Academy of Military Medical Sciences, taking advantage of the limited research data, proposed a compound prescription combining pyrimethamine with dapsone, which, known as "Antimalaria 1", was mainly used for emergency prevention. Soon afterwards in the same year, those experts made persistent efforts and developed the new drugs known as "Antimalaria 2" and "Antimalarial 3" with a longer prevention cycle.

In the late 1960s, China was in a mess. Scientific research, production and culture suffered from unprecedented destruction, and the antimalarial mission also became "insignificant", downgraded from its once "all-important" status. At some point, however, Premier Zhou Enlai instructed researchers to carry out nationwide collaboration for research on drugs to prevent and treat chronic bronchitis, coronary atherosclerotic heart disease and malaria, through combining traditional Chinese and Western medicine. With the joint efforts of experts all around China, a certain level of success in the prevention and treatment of malaria was eventually achieved.

At the time, the General Logistics Department of the PLA sent out invitations to the Scientific and Technological Commission, Ministry of Health, Ministry of Chemical Industry, Commission on Science, Technology, and Industry for National Defense, and the Chinese Academy of Sciences, as well as their affiliated units in fields of scientific research, medical treatment, education, and pharmacy, all of which were expected to cooperate with one another under a unified plan, and jointly undertake the research mission. On May 23, 1967, a national collaboration meeting, organized by the Scientific and Technological Commission and the General Logistics Department of the PLA, attended by the relevant ministries and commissions, subordinate units of the army and the leaders and affiliated units of the relevant provinces, cities, autonomous regions and military regions, was held in Beijing. Due to time urgency and involvement of aid to other countries, the project was simply named "Project 523" after the date of the meeting.

"Project 523" was not just an artemisinin research project; it covered all aspects of malaria prevention and control. This project, lasting for about 13 years, gathered more than 60 scientific research units around China. According to statistics, the number of regular staff participating in the project reached 500–600, and that of participants, with the addition of those involved at different periods, numbered up to 2,000–3,000.

The "Working Team of Project 523" (National Malaria Prevention and Control Drugs Collaborative Research Team) once organized dozens of units from seven major provinces and cities to carry out the joint research. By 1969, more than ten thousand kinds of compounds and medical herbs including *Artemisia annua* L. had been screened, but none of which realized the ideal effect.

> *In January 1969, as invited by Xu Renhe, Deputy President of Guang'anmen Hospital, Academy of Chinese Medical Sciences, the "Working Team of Project 523" visited the Academy of Chinese Medical Sciences. At that critical moment, Tu Youyou, working in the Institute of Chinese Materia Medica and entrusted with antimalarial research, had no idea that her knowledge and practical background obtained from the combination of Chinese traditional and Western medicine would enable the encounter to become one of the brightest glories to China and to the global history of medicine in the future.*

Horrible Malaria

Malaria is an infectious disease that has been threatening human health and life; it is mainly spread by mosquito bites or transfusion of blood with plasmodia. In ancient times, people believed that malaria was caused by miasm, such as water or toxic vapor in swamps; therefore, the English word "malaria" is composed from "Mala" (bad) and "Aria" (air) in Italian.

Reading the yellowed historical materials, it is quite possible to tangibly experience the horrible atmosphere created by the controlling hold of malaria in ancient times.

A Horrible Disease

Malaria is an infectious disease that threatens human health and life; it is mainly spread by mosquito bites or transfusion of blood with plasmodia. In ancient times, people believed that malaria was caused by miasm, such as water or toxic vapor in swamps; therefore, the English word "malaria" is composed from "Mala" (bad) and "Aria" (air) in Italian. Since ancient times, human beings have been suffering from this mosquito-borne infectious disease.

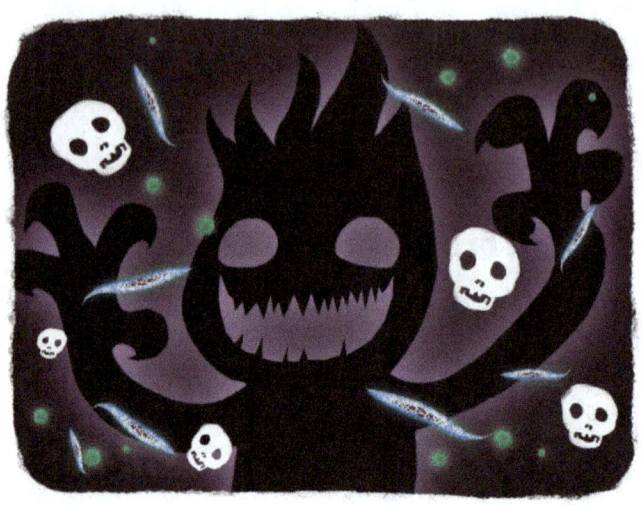

Horrible malaria (drawn by Zhang Linhao).

From the recordings of *Pan Geng Zhong of The Book of History*, a historical document compiled 2490 years ago, we know malaria plagued the Shang Dynasty some 3000 years ago. Thereafter, both Chinese and foreign historical materials have recorded many stories about malaria, fully expressing the horror of the disease.

A Mysterious Leaf

It is said in the Three Kingdoms Period (about 1,800 years ago), Zhuge Liang, Prime Minister of the Kingdom of Shu, led the army to Nanzhong (Southwest of Yunnan Province, Guizhou Province and Sichuan Province, i.e. Southwestern China) to squash the revolt of Meng Huo, leader of local ethnic minorities, who, after several defeats, withdrew to Lushui as suggested by his counselor. Thereafter, Zhuge Liang commanded the army of Shu to cross the Lushui River. It was March and April; toxic miasm gathered and killed most of the 3,000 soldiers who crossed the river. Zhuge Liang, despite being extremely intelligent, had no way to solve the problem.

Fortunately, with the instruction of Fubo General and a brother of Meng Huo, Zhuge Liang ordered each of his soldiers to keep a mysterious leaf in his mouth, thus all their lives were saved. It is believed that what they kept in their mouths were leaves of the well-known *Artemisia annua* L.

A Scary Ballad

In 1300, when China was under the rule of the Yuan Dynasty, Liu Shen, Junior Councilor of Huguang Province, sent an army to conquer Yunnan. The ethnic minorities in Yunnan suffered from the atrocities of Liu's soldiers and when they could bear it no longer, they launched the shocking "Uprising of Eight Hundred Daughters-in-Law". In 1301, 60,000 of Liu's soldiers were trapped in Xishuangbanna, where there was severe malaria, as a result, almost nine out of ten men died before even fighting. As such, the uprising force won a great victory.

At that time, Liu Shen did not know of the scary ballad in Xishuangbanna, "If ten people go to Mengla, nine shall not return home; if one wants to go to Chefonan, he must first buy a coffin; and if one intends to go to Pusaba, he should first let his wife get remarried."

A Bold Inference

Of course, malaria is not exclusive to China. According to historical materials, malaria has had a longer history in the Western world. Over three thousand years ago, the Sumerians, living in Mesopotamia, were extremely fearful of malaria and believed that malaria was a sentence from Nergal, God of Plague, to punish human beings. In 2001, archaeologists from Britain and the United States excavated several bones of children from a tomb belonging to the Ancient Roman period, through gene analysis, they found the clue of malaria infection, and on this basis made a bold inference: The demise of the Ancient Roman Empire probably had something to do with malaria, for there was no drug or method of curing malaria considering the scientific level at that time. Records showed that Galen, a famous physician in Ancient Rome, had failed to discover an effective drug against malaria; instead, Galen, believing that malaria was caused by body fluid imbalance, proposed an assumed treatment method of maintaining balance through bloodletting or purgation. But as proven by modern medical science, bloodletting, just like malaria, may lead to anemia; therefore, "blood-letting therapy" could have actually accelerated the demise of the Ancient Roman Empire.

A Hateful Tyrant

Henry VIII, a well-known King of England, was one of the celebrities killed by malaria. Under his reign, over 70,000 people, including his queen, were killed by him, a terrifying number, considering that in the early 16th century, there were only around 2 million people in England.

One may ask: What did malaria have to do with the homicidal behavior of Henry VIII? According to historical records, Henry VIII was infected with chronic malaria at the age of 30, which, as a recurrent disease, tortured him together with migraine and anabrosis. Some historians believed the reason that Henry VIII repeatedly killed his people was the distortion to his personality caused by the "torment" of malaria.

> *Even now in the 21st century, there are still about 3.3 billion people in 97 countries and regions around the world suffering from the risk of malaria infection, 1.2 billion of whom are under high risk (more than one case of malaria infection in every one thousand people per year). In 2013, it was estimated that there were 198 million people infected with malaria, and 584,000 for whom it was fatal. It seems that the disaster film "directed" by malaria may never come to an end.*

History of the
Antimalarial Fight

Ge Hong, in addition to dividing malaria into six major categories, also provided more than 40 therapeutic methods, which covered various fields of materia medica. To our surprise, the treatment with "Artemisia annua L.", a well-known herb nowadays, was also listed as one of the effective antimalarial methods. It is worth noting that such a method was proposed in the Eastern Jin Dynasty over 1,600 years ago, when science was still extremely backward.

"Since it is a disaster film that may never come to an end, let's try to turn off the projector." Since the appearance of malaria, human beings have been fighting against it. The brave ones, regardless of negative criticism and sacrifice of lives, have been dauntlessly fighting malaria with their own weapons again and again; yet, many of them have failed in the process.

Handbook of Prescriptions for Emergency

In China, an "antimalarial pioneer" began his fight in the Eastern Jin Dynasty. Due to numerous wars, battlefields were hotbeds of various diseases. In turbulent times, there are always heroes. The one worth mentioning here is Ge Hong, a famous medical scientist known as "Xiao Xian Weng" (Supernatural Being), who was second to none in achievements of alchemy and materia medica in that period. In order to let the majority of people master the methods of first aid, especially for meeting emergencies, Ge Hong compiled the medical book *Handbook of Prescriptions for Emergency*, which records therapeutic methods for many diseases, including prescription, acupuncture and manipulation methods.

In the part of "malaria" included in the *Handbook*, Ge Hong, in addition to dividing malaria into six major categories, also provided more than 40 therapeutic methods, which covered various fields of *Materia Medica*. To our surprise, the treatment with "*Artemisia annua* L.", a well-known herb nowadays, was also listed as one of the effective antimalarial methods. It is worth noting that such a method was proposed in the Eastern Jin Dynasty over 1,600 years ago, when science was still extremely backward.

Compendium of Materia Medica

In the Ming Dynasty, Medical Expert Li Shizhen, with his talent, diligence and courage, completed the master work — *Compendium of Materia Medica* — in the field of pharmacy through the practice of "Shen Nong Tast[ing] Hundreds of Herbs". Among the 1,892 kinds of medical herbs in the book, *Artemisia annua* L., as the "antimalarial pioneer", made its appearance again.

Li Shizhen believed radix bupleuri could be used to treat various kinds of malaria, in addition, he also integrated the *Artemisia annua* L. mentioned in his compilation *Shen Nong's Herbal Classic*, that for treating malaria in *Handbook of Prescriptions for Emergency*, and that for treating "malaria cold" through his practice. However, he also recorded another Artemisia herb with different plant morphology, property and efficacy for treating "children's cold", leading to the misidentification with *Artemisia annua*.

A Knocking Brick for the Door of the Qing Dynasty

During the Qing Dynasty, malaria even threatened the life of the emperor. The eight-banner soldiers were unaware that they were carrying plasmodia to Beijing during their triumphant return after the "Revolt of the Three Feudatories". Thereafter, mosquitoes started spreading malaria in Beijing. Emperor Kangxi also became one of those infected.

As recorded in historical materials, Emperor Kangxi suffered from the symptom of "fever alternating with chills", similar to that of malaria. Imperial physicians in the Imperial Academy of Medicine could not provide any effective treatment, for they had not previously encountered such a disease. Therefore, they gathered a group of patients infected with malaria in the palace, and did clinical trials on them. However, they did not find any solution after exhausting all the prescriptions passed down through history. The helpless imperial physicians could do nothing but offer a humble apology, and Emperor Kangxi called upon his people to offer effective prescriptions. Soon enough, countless prescriptions, pills, massage therapy, and even Buddhist scriptures were sent to the Forbidden City. In order to ensure the personal safety of Emperor Kangxi, the four ministers responsible for the mornarch personally consumed the various medicines first before testing of efficacy was done on patients with malaria. Even so, no effective antimalarial method was found.

Thereafter, the common people began worrying about their future given the possible death of Emperor Kangxi, whilst the imperial physicians prepared themselves to pay for their incompetence with death. At a critical juncture, two foreigners in black with a cross and speaking poor Chinese asked to visit Emperor Kangxi; they were missionaries who had served as teachers of Emperor Kangxi and they told the ministers that what Emperor Kangxi was infected with was the fearsome malaria that could be cured with quinine.

Such a suggestion caused an intense debate and the ministers remained skeptical. In clinical trials, however, quinine successfully cured three patients, and the ministers taking quinine also felt fine, which led Emperor Kangxi to firmly believe in the efficacy of quinine. After taking it for a few days, he was completely cured. Later, Emperor Kangxi, disregarding opposition from his ministers, widely introduced quinine into China. Therefore, quinine became the first "knocking brick" for Western powers to knock on the door of the secluded Qing Dynasty.

Legend of Cinchona

Why were the two Western missionaries so confident of curing Emperor Kangxi? In the early 16th century, the magical effect of cinchona was widely known in the distant Americas. There was a legend that a long time ago, an Incan who was suffering from extremely high fever was extremely thirsty, but he could only find a pool of stagnant water after searching in the mountains for a long time. Being completely parched, he decided to drink the water from that pool, for he thought he would die anyway, and afterwards he gently closed his eyes. Unexpectedly, when he opened his eyes a few hours later, he felt completely well. The overjoyed man, wanting to find out the reason for his recovery, attributed it to the uniqueness of that pool of water. Inspired by the tree bent over the pool, he soaked the bark in water and deduced that water soaked with the bark of that tree could cure the disease that he once had. The mysterious tree was known as the cinchona, thereafter, this treatment became a part of folk medicine to cure the symptoms of fever and chills.

In 1630, the wife of Governor of Peru was infected with malaria when she visited Lima. The anxious Governor tried his best to find an effective prescription, but in vain. When he was praying for his dying wife, some Native Americans came to visit him, and cured his wife with a bowl of decoction prepared from the bark of tree named the "tree of life". This led the grateful Governor of Peru to begin re-examining the extraordinary power of the local people. The miraculous "tree of life" was, of course, the cinchona that we are familiar with and quinine is the compound derived from its tree bark.

But the discovery of quinine did not provide peace of mind for long. The strain of malaria that plagued Southeast Asia again in the

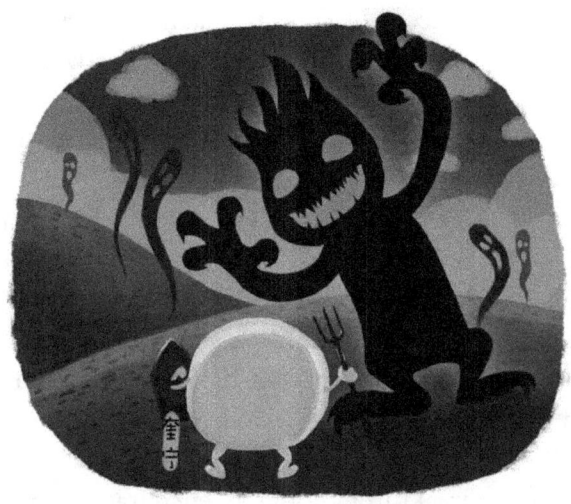

Resistance of malaria to quinine (drawn by Zhang Linhao).

1960s had strong resistance to most quinine-based drugs. As such, the spread of malaria during that epidemic was near impossible.

The Discovery of Ross

Ronald Ross, born in Almora of Uttaranchal, India in 1857, had witnessed the miserable situation of people struggling with malaria since his childhood. In India at that time, millions of people would die of malaria each year; therefore, the local people even called it the "King of Diseases".

Many years later, Ross became a doctor and practiced in London. While examining a woman in Essex, Northeast England one day, he told her that she was infected with malaria. Immediately, she turned pale and fled in panic. Although there was no malaria in Britain at that time, its severity had made it well-known everywhere.

At that moment, Ross suddenly thought of his own experience: in India, he always suffered from various mosquito-borne diseases, so he had started researching on mosquitoes. In the research process, he found that mosquito larvae mainly lived in water, and if the accumulated water was poured away, the number of mosquitoes would be greatly reduced. Just in an instant, he was inspired, and made up his mind to find out the relationship between mosquitoes and malaria.

From 1881 to 1894, Ross travelled tirelessly between Britain and India; not only did he write adventure stories that were popular at the time, he also made time to learn bacteriology and how to use a microscope. In 1895, Ross had an opportunity to discuss the relationship between mosquitoes and malaria with the tropical disease expert Doctor Patrick Manson. They took over the work begun by Laveran, a French doctor, to observe the blood of sailors returning from Africa, and proved that red blood cells could be infected with plasmodia.

Such a major breakthrough greatly encouraged Ross. But when he returned to India in 1895, all the experiments that he conducted ended in failure. Pummeled, he suddenly realized: there might be only one type of mosquitoes carrying the parasite among thousands of species of mosquitoes. Later, he experimented with feeding blood from a malaria patient to the "spot-wing mosquitoes". This patient, named Husein Khan, was offered one copper coin (the currency used in India then) every time he was bitten by a mosquito; he finally accummulated ten copper coins before leaving the laboratory.

Afterwards, Ross immediately killed the mosquito and cut apart its tissues; what was exciting was that he found the malaria parasite in mosquito tissues. In 1898, Ross was dispatched to Kolkata, India, and given a laboratory of his own. Continuing with his experiments, he allowed mosquitoes that had bitten sick birds to bite uninfected birds, resulting in the uninfected ones also becoming infected. Excited, he immediately wrote a letter to Manson, in addition to mentioning the experiments that he conducted on birds, he also described the "germ rods" that he had found on the stomach walls of mosquitoes: the "germ rods", after being placed into the blood cavity, unexpectedly appeared in salivary glands a week later.

At that point, Ross had successfully discovered the complex life cycle of plasmodia. In 1902, he won the Nobel Prize in Physiology or

Medicine with this discovery. Although Ross had picked up on Laveran's work on malaria, he actually won the Nobel Prize five years earlier than Laveran.

> *While Ross had uncovered the nature of production and development of malaria, its therapy was not obviously improved. For the people suffering from malaria, life was both a painstaking struggle and a seemingly interminable wait for the appearance of new antimalarial drugs.*

War and Malaria

The US armed forces suffering from malaria in North Africa and the South Sea Islands were fortunate enough to find a mysterious white tablet from the captured Indonesian soldiers, which inspired American scientists to compound chloroquine, the appearance of which dispelled the fear of malaria.

Natural disasters often occur together with man-made calamities. In the 20th century, human beings suffered from endless pain caused by wars all over the world, which also provided more opportunities for malaria to show its formidable force.

The Battle of Gallipoli

During World War I, the Anglo-French Allied Force endeavoured to land at Gallipoli, unfortunately, they were fiercely beat back by the Turkish army, which caused great losses. This became well-known as the Battle of Gallipoli. In this brutal battle, both sides suffered injuries and deaths numbering some 500,000, with many of the deaths being due to malaria.

It was recorded that both sides stalemated until May. Due to the hot weather, mosquitoes breeded quickly, and there was a large number of wounded soldiers; thereafter, malaria and dysentery plagued the armed forces. After a fierce battle at the end of May, more than 8,000 corpses were left on the battlefield — an area of only several square kilometers. The pervading stink lingering in the air was akin to hovering dark clouds (of malaria). To prevent further spread of malaria, General Birdwood of the Allied Forces, under the dire warning of medical staff, was compelled to order a ceasefire with the Turkish army in order to bury the dead soldiers. During the nine hours of ceasefire on May 24, all surviving soldiers, missionaries, doctors and generals became "mourners".

World War II

During World War II, malaria continued to haunt every battlefield, contributing to the death toll. On battlefields in the east, Japanese soldiers, who had taken part in countless massacres as they marched across China, were similarly massacred by malaria.

The odor of corpses spreading all over China soon became a "cloud of malaria", which slowly extended to every corner of the country. From then on, China, the main eastern battlefield, became one of the warm homes of malaria. The Japanese came to know of quinine and turned to attack the cinchona plantation in Java operated by the Netherlanders, so as to monopolize the source of quinine.

The US armed forces suffering from malaria in North Africa and the South Sea Islands were fortunate enough to find a mysterious white tablet from the captured Indonesian soldiers, which inspired American scientists to compound chloroquine, the appearance of which dispelled the fear of malaria, thus enabling them to start the strategic counter offensive more rapidly.

What was the situation of the US army before the emergence of chloroquine? In April 1942, the Battle of the Philippines was fully underway, and the Japanese army, relying on its powerful naval prowess, launched a general attack on the US-Philippines Allied Force stationed in Bataan. At that time, the surrounded US army had run out of ammunition and food supplies, and soldiers had to hunt monkeys, lizards and snakes for food. 80% of soldiers in the US army were infected with malaria, 75% of whom were also infected with dysentery, and 35% of whom were infected with beriberi. Under the waves of strong attacks by Japanese army, the US-Philippines Allied Force, without any power to resist, was forced to surrender.

The Vietnam War

After World War II, the global war ceased, but malaria continued to plague battlefields around the world.

In 1964, the Vietnam War broke out, and the so-called "invincible" US soldiers were sent to support South Vietnam. Unexpectedly, the largest enemy that they faced was not North Vietnam, but the formidable strain of malaria that was resistant to chloroquine. As recorded, the non-combat loss rate for the US army due to malaria was 3–5 times of the combat loss rate. Malaria, therefore, was named the "single top military medical problem for US armed forces in Vietnam". Certainly, they were unable to find a solution in a short period of time. In 1965,

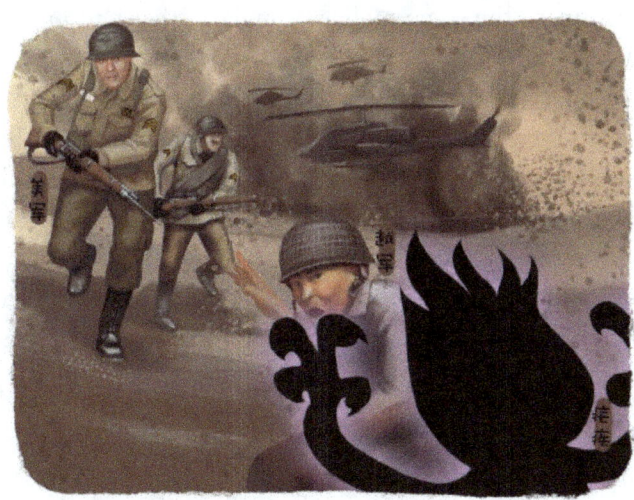

The US army suffered greatly from malaria (drawn by Zhang Linhao).

the annual incidence rate of malaria afflicting the US army in Vietnam reached 50%.

The Vietnamese army could not escape from malaria either. Soldiers infected with malaria would suffer from high fever, headache, vomiting, convulsions, coma, tic, encephaledema, and even death. Moreover, once a soldier was infected with malaria, he had to be transported by two others with a stretcher and escorted by a third one with a gun, thus greatly reducing the efficiency of the march.

The Sequel to Malaria

There was a sequel to malaria in Vietnam, as Jim Manuel, a Vietnam War veteran discovered. One day in the mid-1980s, he went as usual to the Veterans Administration Medical Center in Cedar Rapids, Iowa, for post-traumatic stress disorder (PTSD) counseling. When he learnt that there was a study being done on veterans who had contracted malaria in Vietnam, he was intrigued and agreed to participate.

A big problem was revealed: testing by the neurologist revealed a 30-point drop in his IQ from his military induction exam and an abnormal electroencephalograph. He finally found the root of his nightmares, his uncontrollable temper, and his frequent frustration and depression — the same malice of malaria that had once tortured Henry VIII.

He recalled his suffering from malaria at a military camp in Vietnam a dozen years ago. Manuel was 19 when he volunteered for military service in November 1965. Ten months later, he found himself deep in the Central Highlands of Vietnam near the Cambodian border, one of 158 men in an Army Infantry Company. From October 1966 to September 1967, he estimated his company lost 25 to 30 men, with one instance of 11 men in just one day. Unfortunately, he was infected with cerebral malaria like others, fortunately, he remained alive.

> *Humankind restarted the fight against malaria and the exploration of new drugs after realizing the fact that "malaria is perhaps more horrific than war".*

The Launch of Antimalarial Research

In July 1969, i.e. in summer when malaria was most severe, the Office of "Project 523" dispatched Tu Youyou, Lang Linfu and Yu Yagang to work in Hainan Province. Tu Youyou, after consulting with her husband Li Tingzhao, reluctantly sent their eldest daughter to a full-time childcare facility, and then set out for Hainan Province with two other colleagues.

After receiving the appeal of Vietnam, Chairman Mao, who had once been infected with malaria during wartime, was determined to help. To him, malaria not only affected that war, but also concerned the health of the Chinese people. With the launch of "Project 523" and the development of antimalarial work, the incidence of malaria in China was reduced, but no ideal results were gained in the field of developing efficient, quick-acting, and long-acting antimalarial drugs.

Collection of Antimalarial Prescriptions

In 1969, Tu Youyou was 39 years old. In view of her solid knowledge of Chinese and Western medicine and outstanding research capability, she was appointed as leader of the antimalarial research team. Initially, she was the only member of the team. Confronting her at the time was a challenging task: scientific research had stagnated, the equipment available was old and resources were lacking. The situation was worse than compared to a decade before.

The book *Chemistry of Chinese Medicinal Herb Ingredients* compiled by Lin Qishou and many past research on extraction of effective chemical components from herbs provided Tu with some inspiration on getting started. Realizing that there must be truths in traditional Chinese medicine, she started studying the *Compendium of Materia Medica*, collecting and sorting through ancient medical books, looking up folk prescriptions and consulting with old specialists.

During that period, she looked through a large number of individual herbs and compound prescriptions with records and clinical practices from her predecessors; collected and sorted many ancient medical books besides the *Compendium of Materia Medica*; read all the letters from people after the founding of the Academy; and consulted with the well-known old doctors hired throughout China. From the expansive beach of medical knowledge, Tu managed to pick up many beautiful shells. The famous traditional Chinese doctor Pu Fuzhou recommended compound prescriptions "Lei Ji San" and "Sheng San Zi", and another famous physician Yue Meizhong recommended "Mu Zei Jian" and "Guizhi Baihu Tang".

In two months, Tu painstakingly immersed herself in the wisdom of traditional Chinese medicine, carefully selecting and collecting more than 2,000 herbal, animal and mineral prescriptions for both oral administration and external use. Finally, she completed the *Collection of Antimalarial Prescriptions* which contained more than 640 prescriptions; it was printed and sent to the Office of "Project 523" in April 1969.

The Indistinct *Artemisia Annua* L.

When researchers at that time read through this collection, they did not notice that *Artemisia annua* L., so well-known in antimalarial circles years later, had been frequently mentioned.

On page 15, there is such a record:

Prescription: *Artemisia annua* L., five qian (about 25g) to half a jin (250g)

Directions for Use: Extract juice by crushing, decoct with water or mix the grinded powder with hot water.

Sources: Fujian, Guizhou, Yunnan, Guangxi, Hunan, and Jiangxi.

Remarks: There are also other methods of preparation from various regions such as: 3 liang (150g) of *Artemisia annua* L. and 3 liang (150g) of false sesame, take decocted with water, this is said to have good curative effect.

These prescriptions containing *Artemisia annua* L. had been silently absorbed by Tu Youyou's mind and integrated into her experiments, although at the time her efforts were focused on finding herbal medicine that could treat the bergseife-induced side effect of vomiting.

Firing the First Shot at Malaria

In May 1969, Tu started preparing Chinese medicinal herb water extract and ethanol extract, which were then sent to the Academy of Military Medical Sciences (hereinafter referred to as "236") as part of the screening of antimalarial drugs. By late June, Tu had sent more than 50 specimens in total, among which, pepper extract seemed to have the best effect: its inhibition ratio to rodent model plasmodia (the ratio of inhibiting cell growth of plasmodia) reached 84%.

In July 1969, i.e. in summer when malaria was most severe, the Office of "Project 523" dispatched Tu Youyou, Lang Linfu and Yu Yagang to work in Hainan Province. Tu Youyou, after consulting with her husband Li Tingzhao, reluctantly sent their eldest daughter to a full-time childcare facility, and then set out for Hainan Province with two other colleagues. They took two specimens with high rodent malaria inhibition rate (from screening in the first half of the year), namely pepper and a mixture of chili and alums, to conduct observations on their clinical curative effects. They had great expectations, unfortunately the outcome of their trial was not satisfactory: Although several specimens prepared on the basis of pepper and a mixture of chili and alums achieved the rodent malaria inhibition ratio of above 80%, they failed to completely eliminate the plasmodia and could only improve the symptoms of patients with malaria.

While she was granted the "Five-Good Member Title" by the Guangdong "Project 523" Office for her work on this trial, Tu Youyou was nevertheless discouraged by this failure.

In 1970, the research team began focusing on in-depth study of pepper. From February to September of the same year, Tu and her colleagues successively sent more than 120 specimens prepared with various extracts and mixtures for testing. The test results seemed to declare the "death" of pepper in the antimalarial war: its titer, through separation and extraction, could not be improved; even though it could be increased after adjusting the component ratio, the effect was far inferior to chloroquine.

After arduous discussions, Tu Youyou and her colleagues realized they had to change their focus. Thereafter, they expanded the scope of screening; Tu was responsible for screening medical herbs, while Yu Yagang was responsible for screening medicines from mineral and animal sources.

A Way Out

The mammoth task assigned by "236", as well as the fact that the Institute of Chinese Materia Medica was ill-equipped to carry out antimalarial activity detection at that time posed difficulties for Tu Youyou. Tu's team, with over 30 screened specimens including the ethanol extract that could achieve 68% of plasmodia inhibition rate, regrettably stopped the screening of antimalarial medicines only one year after firing their first shot at malaria.

"Opportunity knocks on the doors of the prepared", Tu Youyou did not have to wait too long. In 1971, the Vietnam War entered its most brutal phase, and malaria also appeared in South China, resulting in great demand for antimalarial drugs both at home and abroad. From May 22 to June 1, in accordance with the instruction of the State Council (71) Document Release (29) issued by the State Council and Central Military Commission, the National Malaria Control and Lead Research Team held a malaria control and research symposium in Guangzhou. The symposium summarized the domestic antimalarial research situation and proposed the emphasis and requirements of afive-year plan of malaria prevention and control work. During the symposium, Premier Zhou sent a telegram, making an important instruction to strengthen the prevention and control of falciparum malaria in tropical regions. The antimalarial movement was revived in China: research teams on malaria prevention and control integrating Chinese traditional medicine with Western medicine, preclinical medicine with clinical medicine, and acupuncture with medicinal treatment all actively responded to the Premier's call.

At that time, a leader of the Ministry of Health commented that the work of "Project 523" on traditional Chinese medicine should only progress and not regress. Tu Youyou also participated in the symposium. Her work gained approval from the senior leadership present at the meeting and the Academy of Chinese Medical Sciences, "serving again as ordered", was tasked to continue its research into traditional Chinese medicine for prevention and treatment of malaria. The leaders allowed Tu Youyou to set up a research team consisting of four members: Tu Youyou was responsible for the overall work, Lang Linfu was responsible for establishing the animal models of rodent malaria and simian malaria, and the other two members were Liu Jufu and Zhong Yurong. Although there were only four members in the team, they worked quite hard and could screen two batches of specimens each week.

On July 16, 1971, Tu Youyou, leading her companions, continued to make progress on the long and arduous road of screening antimalarial medical herbs. By early September 1971, over 200 aqueous extract and alcohol extract specimens prepared on the basis of more than 100 medical herbs had been screened on the laboratory table. Through screening of over 380 specimens prepared on the basis of more than

200 medical herbs, the team narrowed their focus onto *Artemisia annua* L. But after several rounds of experiment, *Artemisia annua* L. was a disappointment: its inhibition ratio to plasmodia could only reach around 40% at the highest, and only around 12% at the lowest.

Herbs screening record of Tu's team in 1971.

The experiment results seemed to declare the termination of Artemisia annua L., and also pour a pot of cold water on Tu Youyou's aspiration.

Inspiration and Success

At some point in time, she read, "take a handful of Artemisia annua L., soak in water of two liters, extrude juice, and take it all," recorded in Prescriptions for Curing Malaria Chills and Fever No. 16, Vol. III, Handbook of Prescriptions for Emergency. Suddenly, she seemed to see lightning pierce through dark clouds, a strong wind blew away the dense fog, and light appeared from darkness. A fantastic idea came to her mind.

Studying the Ancient Books of Traditional Chinese Medicine

With the poor performance of *Artemisia annua* L. in the model test of rodent malaria, Tu fell into self doubt: Could it be that *Artemisia annua* L. was unable to treat malaria? Could it be that what was recorded in ancient books was unauthentic? Could it be that the experimental scheme was unreasonable? The huge pressure on top of her tireless experiments began to take a toll on her health.

Artemisia annua L., so promising initially in eyes of Tu and her companions, seemed to withdraw from the antimalarial stage, returning to play the role of a traditional herb for clearing deficient heat.

"Patience and persistence, although difficult, gradually leads to success"; indeed, as far as Tu Youyou and her companions were concerned, there was no "failure". She started reading the ancient books of traditional Chinese medicine once more.

Relying on the knowledge accumulated from the Traditional Chinese Medicine Training Workshop for Western Medical Doctors and the experience of compiling the *Collection of Antimalarial Prescriptions*, Tu Youyou was clearly aware that *Artemisia annua* L. had been taken as medicine; although there were different records, it was mainly prepared through boiling. In her mind, she began sorting through all the differences of *Artemisia annua* L. in *Shen Nong's Herbal Classic*, the *Handbook of Prescriptions for Emergency* and the *Compendium of Materia Medica*.

With further reflection, Tu Youyou only strengthened her confidence in *Artemisia annua* L.

Inspiration Piercing through Dark Clouds

Tu Youyou carefully read the ancient books word by word, and tried to understand each detail. At some point in time, she read, "take a handful of *Artemisia annua* L., soak in water of two liters, extrude juice, and take it all," recorded in *Prescriptions for Curing Malaria Chills and Fever No. 16, Vol. III, Handbook of Prescriptions for Emergency*. Suddenly, she seemed to see lightning pierce through dark clouds, a strong wind blew away the dense fog, and light appeared from darkness. A fantastic idea came to her mind:

The less prominent antimalarial efficacy of *Artemisia annua* L. could be caused by high temperature or enzymolysis. The antimalarial method of *Artemisia annua* L might require the breakthrough of the historical tradition.

In the countless experiments conducted previously, the team had employed various methods of discovering antimalarial substances, however, most of them relied on increasing temperature. The reason why the ancients could successfully treat malaria with juice extruded from *Artemisia annua* L. was that they had inadvertently avoided the factor of high temperature. Perhaps, artemisinin might be harmed by

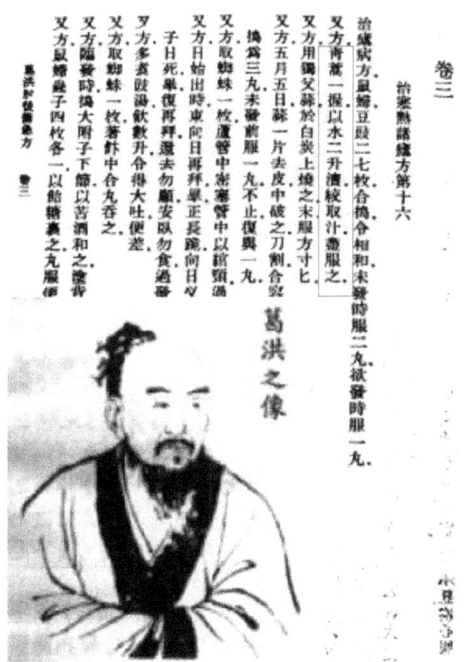

Record in *Prescriptions for Curing Malaria Chills and Fever No. 16, Vol. III, Handbook of Prescriptions for Emergency*: Take a handful of *Artemisia annua* L., soak in water of two liters, extrude juice, and take it all.

high temperature? If it was extracted in another way, would it then become effective?

> *Tu Youyou, led by her inspiration, hesitated no further and went to the bedstand again. Seemingly, the inspiration ignited by "take a handful of Artemisia annua L., soak in water of two liters, extrude juice, and take it all," would never be extinguished. Under the guidance of this thought, Tu Youyou continued moving forward …*

Inspiration and Success   55

Specimen 191

Long-term exposure to the harmful ether and other organic solvents had affected the health of many in the team, with Tu herself being infected with toxic hepatitis; however, they were too industrious to take care of themselves. Besides, other scientific researchers in China at that time also put the nation and collective first. For them, the foremost priority was: self-sacrifice for the collective good.

The New Extraction Scheme

"As guided by ancient books, the key to extracting artemisinin is temperature. If we extract it at a low temperature, we may achieve success". It was not long before Tu Youyou started developing a new extraction scheme.

Beginning from September 1971, the research team, under the leadership of Tu Youyou, meticulously thought through and redesigned a new scheme for extracting the active ingredients of *Artemisia annua* L. They selected the leaves of mature Beijing *Artemisia annua* L. that had been picked in autumn and conducted experiments in turn with various methods.

The decoction extract and ethanol extract turned to be invalid in the rodent malaria pharmacological experiments; the extract obtained through ethanol cold soak, with temperature controlled at 60°C during concentration, had a certain effect in the rodent malaria experiment, but it had no effect when the temperature was too high. The extract obtained through ether reflux cold soak showed a quite high titer and stable effect in the rodent malaria experiment.

In *Artemisia annua L. and Artemisinin-based Drugs*, the only work of Tu Youyou published by Chemical Industry Press in 2009, there is such a description, "It shall be particularly noted that during extraction of artemisinin, the key to success is to control the temperature under 60°C. But monomer artemisinin obtained through separation can maintain stable antimalarial efficacy even after being boiled for half an hour or placed in reflux of ethanol for 4h."

Specimen 191

Countless sleepless nights passed. On October 4, 1971, Tu Youyou and her colleagues in the research team were pleasantly surprised to finally

Tu's experimental record, recording the use of *Artemisia annua* L. for Experiment No. 191 with the plasmodia inhibition ratio of 100%.

obtain the result that they had been looking for in the antimalarial experiment on ether neutral extract from Specimen 191: the extract realized a 100% inhibition ratio to plasmodia with lower toxic and side effects and higher antimalarial efficacy!

Their experimental procedures can be summarized as follows: First place the treated ends of *Artemisia annua* L. leaves in ether for cold soak, in this way, the components of the leaves would slowly dissolve in ether, which would become the ether extract after clearing the dregs; then further heat the extract, for the concentration of effective antimalarial ingredients was very low; finally, the concentrated ether extract with efficacy can be obtained.

Due to the large dose during ether extraction and its toxicity, Tu's team separated concentrated ether extract with sodium hydroxide solution of 2%, thus obtaining the neutral extract and acidic extract. Then they carried out targeted experiments on both types of solutions. As showed in experiments: the acidic extract was ineffective with strong toxicity, and the neutral extract was the truly effective extract, which was the *Artemisia annua* L. ether neutral extract, also known as "ether neutral extract".

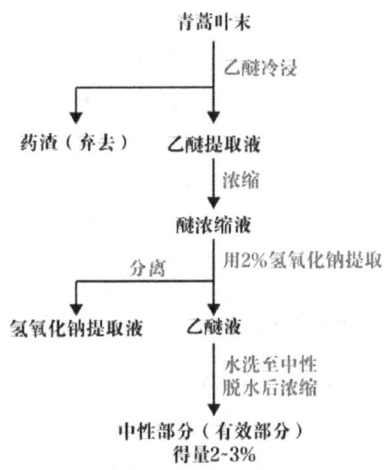

Flowchart of extracting active antimalarial ingredients from *Artemisia annua* L.

Ether with Low Boiling Point

Why is ether suitable for use to extract the effective antimalarial ingredients from *Artemisia annua* L.? The reason is that ether is a colorless, transparent and volatile liquid with acrid odor. Under standard atmospheric pressure, its boiling point is 34.6°C. Due to its low boiling point, the highest temperature that will be reached when heating to prepare the concentrated ether extract is only 34.6°C, which, being far lower than 60°C, would not destroy the effective antimalarial ingredient in the solution. In addition, ether extraction has another advantage: fewer ingredients of the ends of the leaves would dissolve in ether, so there are fewer impurities in ether extract, which is more conducive to purification.

At that time, the research team worked under poor experimental conditions; in order to get more *Artemisia annua* L. ether extract as quickly as possible, they conducted experiments with seven large water vats in replacement of extracting containers in the laboratory. There was neither a ventilation system nor experimental protection equipment in the laboratory; Tu and her colleagues conducted experiments with only gauze masks. Long-term exposure to the harmful ether and other organic solvents affected the health of many in the team, with Tu herself being infected with toxic hepatitis; however, they were too industrious to take care of themselves. Besides, other scientific researchers in China at that time also put the nation and collective first. For them, the foremost priority was: self-sacrifice for the collective good.

Research on *Artemisia annua* L.

Tu's team, before obtaining the effective *Artemisia annua* L. extract, had conducted a large amount of research on identifying and screening *Artemisia annua* L. They found that immature *Artemisia annua* L. contains no artemisinin; only the leaves of *Artemisia annua* L. (and not stalks or roots) have the antimalarial function, with the tender tips of leaves containing the most active ingredients. The best picking time is autumn, for in this season, *Artemisia annua* L. do not bloom and their leaves are the most flourishing. The leaves should be used in the same year they are picked, for the content of active ingredients may be reduced with increase of storage time.

> *The antimalarial research on Artemisia annua L., after three years of twists and turns, had finally achieved a phased victory. During the research, many animals, especially laboratory rats, had played important roles.*

Experiments on Laboratory Rats

Healthy laboratory rats of weight 18–22g were first selected, blood was drawn from the ones infected with malaria, and then 1×10^7 plasmodias was injected into the abdominal cavity of each healthy rat. 24 hours later, ether neutral extract was then injected into the stomachs of laboratory rats, thus beginning their "antimalarial journey".

In the process of drug research, each drug obtained in the laboratory should undergo pharmacological experiments before clinical trials, to verify whether it is active, effective or toxic. The preparation of artemisinin also underwent such a process: After extracting the active ingredient from *Artemisia annua* L. with ether, or obtaining the ether neutral extract through separating the ether extract of *Artemisia annua* L., pharmacological experiments would immediately be conducted on laboratory rats to preliminarily judge the effectiveness and toxicity of what had been obtained in the laboratory. As such, the rats played the role of judge, the success of testing on rats determined whether the process could be considered to have achieve initial success.

Pharmacodynamic Study

Healthy laboratory rats of weight 18–22g were first selected, blood was drawn from the ones infected with malaria, and then 1×10^7 plasmodias was injected into the abdominal cavity of each healthy rat. 24 hours later, ether neutral extract was then injected into the stomachs of laboratory rats, thus beginning their "antimalarial journey".

A few minutes later, a few hours later… a long period of time later, the lovely laboratory rats watched her with curious eyes, many even ran around happily. Tu conducted physical examinations for them in haste, and found that they were quite healthy.

This process was conducted repeatedly over three days. Researchers drew blood from the tails of laboratory rats 24 hours after the last injection of plasmodia, to observe the inhabitation situation of plasmodia. The experimental results showed that all plasmodia in the rats' bodies had disappeared. The success of the rodent malaria experiment represented the first step towards the team's goal for the research on artemisinin.

Soon afterwards, the research team conducted a simian malaria experiment with simians as the experimental targets. The experimental results showed that the neutral part of artemisinin also had an obvious antimalarial function to simian malaria.

The Safety Experiment

First, researchers selected healthy laboratory rats and observed them for three days after a one-time injection of plasmodia, to calculate the median lethal dose and other data. The larger the median lethal dose, the safer the drug. Through such an experiment, Tu Youyou calculated that the median lethal dose of ether neutral extract was 7,425 mg/kg. Briefly, for every kilogram of extract, the concentration had to be 7,425 mg in order for half of the rats population tested to be killed. Therefore, the experiment showed that the neutral extract was relatively safe.

Later, the research team also conducted cardiac toxicity experiments on laboratory rats, cats, and dogs; liver toxicity experiments on 13 healthy dogs; kidney toxicity experiments on ten healthy dogs; and pathological examination on eight dogs in two batches.

Tu Youyou brimmed with confidence. The experimental results had proven her conjecture, and all animals had safely undergone the experiments. The results also showed that ether neutral extract had no obvious impact on other visceral organs, except for slight or transient impact on liver transaminase vigor of only a few animals.

Laboratory rats, dogs, simians and other animals played important roles in the pharmacological experiments and safety experiments conducted by Tu's team; to this day, many of them continue to be important experimental subjects in domestic and foreign drug research. They have made great sacrifices for human health and deserve our reverence, compassion and gratitude.

Personally Testing Efficacy

"Let's organize a drug trial. I plan to conduct it by gradually increasing the dosage. I will go first, so now we need another two participants; would anyone like to join me?" In that instant, the excited chatter in the meeting room dissolved into utter silence. "Since no one disagrees, let's just do it!"

Not Giving Up

A pre-clinical dog malaria drug test was conducted on the ether neutral extract soon after its discovery, and one dog had a toxic reaction.

The antimalarial safety of ether neutral extract was questioned, but Tu's team believed its safety could be guaranteed, as proved by all the previous animal toxicity tests that they had carried out; in addition, there was no record of toxicity of *Artemisia annua* L. in ancient books of traditional Chinese medicine over millennia. Many researchers believed however that hidden toxicity might not be found during extraction of the ether neutral extract and building of the rodent malaria model. Furthermore, others even suggested restudying pepper.

The experiments came to a deadlock and artemisinin had to face its moment of destiny.

It was midnight, the members of the team were in the midst of designing experimental schemes and discussing the details, Tu Youyou, who had been listening for a long while, suddenly said in a firm voice:

"I think we should not give up on *Artemisia annua* L."

"We must ensure it is benign to humans, we must not deny the value of *Artemisia annua* L. with just one negative case."

Taking the Lead for a Personal Drug Trial

"Let's organize a drug trial. I plan to conduct it by gradually increasing the dosage. I will go first, so now we need another two participants; would anyone like to join me?" In that instant, the excited chatter in the meeting room dissolved into utter silence. "Since no one disagrees, let's just do it!"

Personal drug trial, for an expert in the field of pharmacognosy, effectively demonstrates "trust in one's personally made drug". At that time, Tu Youyou did not consider too much, she only wanted to be the first to find out whether artemisinin was effective; and only a personal drug trial would enable her to truly experience the drug that she had personally made.

With the approval of her superiors, the first batch of participants consisted of three members: Tu Youyou, Lang Linfu and Yue Fengxian. In July 1972, they moved to Dongzhimen Hospital which was affiliated to Beijing University of Chinese Medicine. This trial was termed "Exploratory Drug Trial". In order to ensure its safety, the research team determined to set

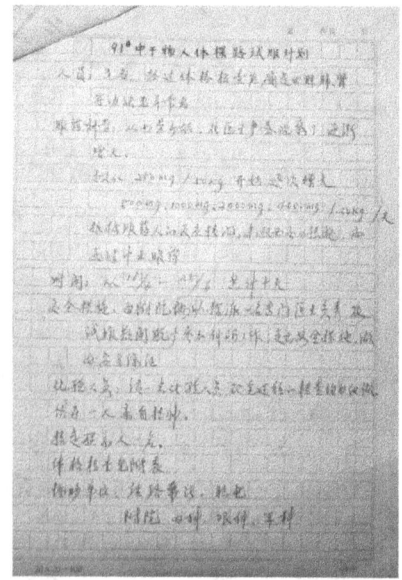

Plan of the "Exploratory Drug Trial".

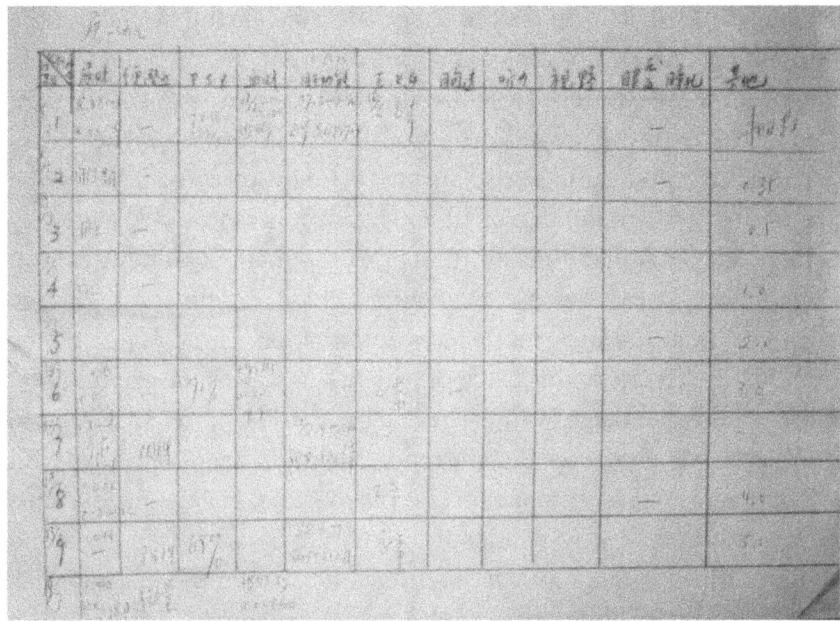

Record of Tu Youyou during the drug trial.

the initial dose as 0.35 g per person. Under the strict monitoring of the hospital, the dose was gradually increased: 0.35 g, 0.5 g, 1.0 g, 2.0 g, 3.0 g, 4.0 g and 5.0 g; they took it once a day and continued taking it for seven days. The result: there was no obvious toxic and side effects from the ether neutral extract to the human body.

Tu Youyou was not exactly in the best of health at the time, and her daughters were still young; however, she charged ahead regardless of her safety for the sake of scientific undertaking. Shi Yigong, Vice President of Tsinghua University commented on her decision: "In the context of her environment, it must have been hard to do such a thing. When scientists experiment on themselves, it is a clear indication of dedication and sacrifice."

More Clinical Trials

In August 1972, with the prepared drugs, Tu Youyou went to Changjiang Malaria Area in Hainan Province with the medical team of the Academy of Chinese Medical Sciences, to carry out clinical studies. Taking the flexibility of clinical dosage schemes into account, and in order to fully demonstrate the efficacy of artemisinin, they quickly organized patients to participate in the second drug trial. Five patients were selected as participants to take a dose of 3.0 g twice a day, for three days. In the pre-trial, in-trial and post-trial periods, researchers would respectively conduct ECG examination, liver function examination, kidney function examination, chest fluoroscopy, routine blood examination, routine urine examination, and routine feces examination. Three days later, the examination results of this batch of patients, as well as the examination results of the first batch (which she had been part of), were reported to Tu Youyou. When she opened the report, her right hand trembling with excitement, she saw what she had been expecting: For the five patients in Hainan Province, the results of the routine blood examination and routine urine examination were normal after taking the drug; kidney functions were in the normal range; urea nitrogen was normal; chest fluoroscopy and ECG examination were normal during and after drug consumption; there was no obvious change in blood pressure; fundus oculi was normal and the vision did not obviously change as compared to the pre-trial reading; body temperature and pulse were normal; and there were no clinical symptoms in the respiratory system, urinary system, and central nervous system. There was only one toxic and side effect: a slight manifestation in the digestive tract, with two patients who suffered from abdominal pain one hour after taking the drug. Nevertheless, it was not severe, and later self-resolved without treatment.

The results of the human drug trial showed that the neutral extract containing artemisinin had no obvious influence on other visceral organs, except for a slight or transient impact on liver transaminase vigor of only a few animals.

In the malaria area in Hainan Province, Tu Youyou and her colleagues eventually completed a total of 21 clinical antimalarial observations. They selected 11 tertian malaria patients, 9 falciparum malaria patients, and 1 patient of mixed infection, all of whom, suffering from persistent fevers of 40°C, were miraculously healed a few days later, with plasmodia in their bodies substantially eliminated. Compared with the slow efficacy of chloroquine, artemisinin was more superior in efficacy. Such a result certainly gave Tu Youyou and other researchers more confidence in artemisinin.

Some time later, the trial was repeated on nine patients at the 302 Military Hospital of China, with excellent results.

In August 1973, another summer season with high incidence of malaria, Tu Youyou, armed with artemisinin monomer purified from effective parts of *Artemisia annua* L., went to the Changjiang Malaria Area in Hainan Province again to carry out clinical studies. Due to the problem of systole (heart chamber contraction) that some patients had before the trial, the number of participants was reduced to 8 from 14. Nevertheless, the trial was very successful.

> *Tu Youyou could finally relax, she recalled the day of October 4, 1971, almost two years ago, when she found that Specimen 191 could achieve a 100% inhibition ratio to rodent malaria plasmodia. At that time, she did not expect that the scientific community would set up a monument for the discovery, nor that numerous researchers with noble aspirations in pharmacognosy and Chinese medicine would gather in front of such a monument.*

Antimalarial Symphony

It seems hard to imagine now, if not for the persistence of Tu Youyou, when artemisinin, the drug curing millions of people each year, would have been discovered. We can only guess at best, the amount of effort on the part of Tu Youyou and her colleagues in their research.

The Prologue

A meeting was held in Nanjing on March 8, 1972, before the drug trial. At the meeting, Tu Youyou, in high and vigorous spirits, stepped up to the rostrum and made the report *Research on Antimalarial Chinese Herbs Guided by Mao Zedong Thought* on behalf of her team.

In the report, she cited a lot of facts and experimental data to show the scientific value and effectiveness of artemisinin to treat malaria; more importantly, in addition to the advanced scientific techniques, her presentation also made clear her commendable spirit of scientific enquiry in research:

> *... It was not always smooth for us to screen an effective antimalarial drug in the laboratory, but a fumbling process requiring trial and error, repeated practice and constant improvement.*

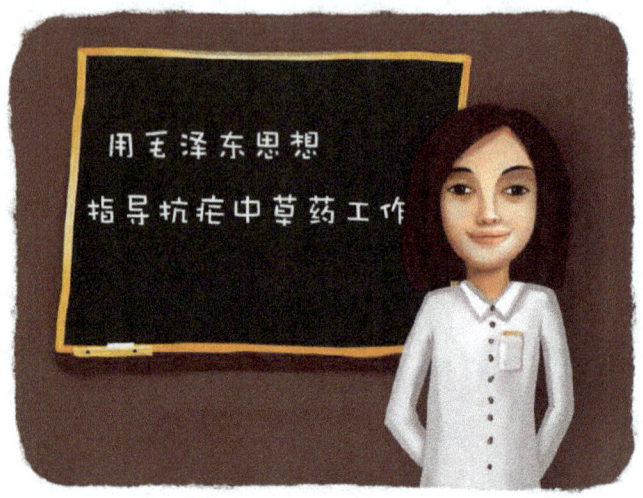

Tu Youyou's report at the Nanjing meeting (drawn by Zhang Linhao).

... The instruction of "practice, recognition, re-practice, and re-recognition" made by Chairman Mao greatly inspired and enlightened us, and encouraged us to overcome the "failure" in screening. As it turns out, "A correct understanding would always be achieved through repetition from substance to spirit and then from spirit to substance, i.e. from practice to understanding and then from understanding to practice".

... We haven't done enough, we have just done the preliminary work, and the laboratory work must be closely combined with clinical work. For a drug, clinical trial is the largest challenge.

What Tu said at the meeting inspired many to become enthusiastic about antimalarial work. A nationwide fever for antimalarial research and treatment began, many experts and scholars were greatly encouraged by the speech; they believed they could made similar achievements like Tu Youyou. Under the direction of the "523" Office, more and more researchers started engaging in antimalarial research.

The Setback

After the Nanjing meeting, Tu Youyou encountered the biggest setback on her journey of antimalarial research: her laboratory caught fire, destroying a lot of data. Nevertheless, Tu, even with such a heavy blow dealt to her, was determined to continued the research, and led the research team to restore the original data and experimental achievements, working tirelessly, day and night.

It seems hard to imagine now, if not for the persistence of Tu Youyou, when artemisinin, the drug curing millions of people each year, would have been discovered. We can only guess at best, the amount of effort on the part of Tu Youyou and her colleagues in their research. In order not to miss the best experimental period of the year, they prepared *Artemisia annua* L. ether extract with large water vats to meet the dosage demand of follow-up clinical trials.

The Upsurge

At the "Malaria Prevention and Treatment Research Conditions Exchange Meeting" held on November 5, 1972, Tu Youyou made a special introduction of antimalarial research with *Artemisia annua* L. At the National "523" Meeting held in Beijing on November 17, 1972, Tu delivered a summary of effective antimalarial efficacy of all 30 cases for the first time, which was affirmed by other participants. As a result, the status of the Institute of Chinese Materia Medica, Academy of Chinese Medical Sciences was gradually elevated. Antimalarial research on *Artemisia annua* L. became popular once again around China.

Subsequently, the active involvement of various parties greatly advanced the progress of antimalarial work. Shandong Province and Yunnan Province willingly served as pioneers, the Institutes of Chinese Medicine in both provinces respectively wrote to the Institute of Chinese Materia Medica, Academy of Chinese Medical Sciences, to ask for further confirmation of the variety of *Artemisia annua* L., to facilitate learning about its type, clinical, toxic and side effects, etc. Carrying out research in full swing, the Shandong Provincial Institute of Materia Medica, in succession to the Shandong Institute of Parasitic Diseases, became the second production unit, and the Yunnan Provincial Institute of Materia Medica became the third production unit of artemisinin.

Exchanges and cooperation among various research units increased. From autumn to winter in 1973, the persons in charge of the "523" Office and Institute of Chinese Materia Medica successively went to Yunnan Province and Shandong Province, to learn about their antimalarial situation.

From February 28 to March 1, 1974, the Academy of Chinese Medical Sciences, under the auspices of the "523 Office", held a "National Artemisinin Antimalarial Collaboration Meeting". After the meeting, relevant information from artemisinin research laboratories under the Institute of Chinese Materia Medica, Academy of Chinese Medical Sciences was disclosed. In addition to offering detailed introduction to the public, the laboratories also allowed public visits, thus allowing more people to develop greater understanding of the antimalarial research. Later, the much encouraged scientific research community launched a dramatic "antimalarial storm", thus creating an opportunity for nationwide collaboration.

Subsequently, the "antimalarial team" in China gradually developed and grew stronger. In addition to the previously mentioned Shandong Province and Yunnan Province, other provinces including Sichuan, Guangxi, and Guangdong also participated in the research; their joint efforts took antimalarial research to a peak. In 1975, the Traditional Chinese Medicine University of Guangzhou participated in the work, expanding the capacity for clinical validation of artemisinin-based drugs, and then it became the sixth production unit of artemisinin. As recorded in the data of the Artemisinin Appraisal Meeting held in 1978, more than 40 units participated in the antimalarial research, and a total of ten provinces, municipalities and autonomous regions participated in the clinical research; a total of 6,555 cases and 2,099 artemisinin preparations were verified. This high number of cases is rare even in new medicine research nowadays.

At that moment, the single antimalarial spark kindled by Tu Youyou finally became a great fire. Following her direction, researchers across China made their own contributions to the same objective and a glorious antimalarial career, no matter what their positions were.

From Crystal to Drug

In 1972, the team, for the first time, extracted effective antimalarial monomer from Artemisia annua L., which was then named artemisinin. Working around the clock, they successfully isolated over 100 g of artemisinin for subsequent clinical antimalarial tests and chemical structure identification.

Extracting Antimalarial Monomer

When ether neutral extract was successfully extracted, Tu's team immediately started extracting the antimalarial monomer.

In the field of traditional Chinese medicine and pharmacy, there are mainly three methods of extraction: the solvent method, steam distillation method and sublimation method, each of which, however, seemed unable to individually extract artemisinin crystals. The extract gained through one of the three methods could not be directly used, and the active ingredient had to be separated several times, to finally determine its active ingredient.

Tu's team designed an experimental scheme on the basis of improvement of previous separating experiments: First mix ether neutral extract with polyamide, infiltrate with 47% ethanol, and conduct decompress concentration for the liquid gained; then extract the concentrated solution with ether again, and conduct slica column chromatography for the extract. Later, they gained two kinds of oil through eluting with petroleum ether: yellow oil and orange oil; and then gained two kinds of white needle crystals and one kind of yellow oil through eluting again with 10% ethyl acetate-petroleum ether. Through determination, the crystals were respectively named Arteannuin A and artemisinin. Finally, a kind of white square crystal and black oily matter were gained through eluting with 15% ethyl acetate-petroleum ether, and the white square crystal was then named as Arteannuin B.

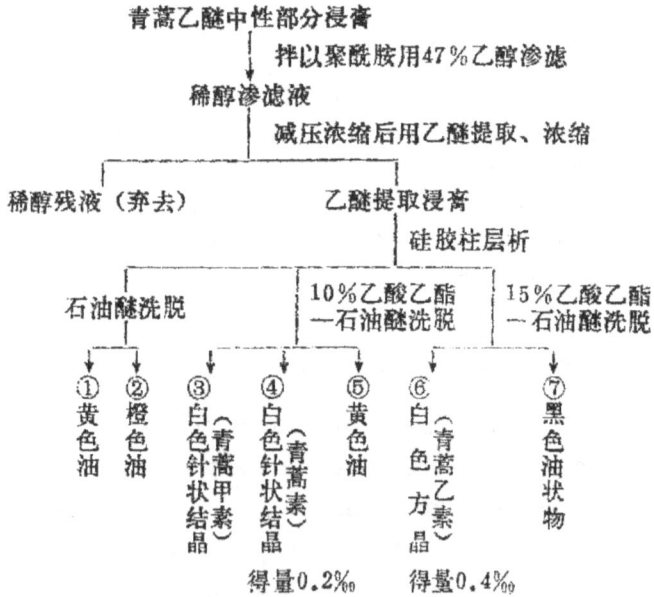

Ether neutral extract separation process.

In later studies, the researchers found Arteannuin B could also play a certain role: when artemisinin was mixed with equivalent Arteannuin B, it could still eliminate plasmodia even when its dose was reduced by half, which proved the precious value of Arteannuin B.

Final Discovery of Artemisinin

Tu's team separately carried out rodent malaria model experiments with products gained through elution. The experimental results showed that the separated yellow oily matter, Arteannuin A and Arteannuin B were invalid and only artemisinin could eliminate all plasmodia in rodent malaria models. In 1972, the team, for the first time, extracted effective antimalarial monomer from *Artemisia annua* L., which was then named artemisinin. Working around the clock, they successfully isolated over 100 g of artemisinin for subsequent clinical antimalarial tests and chemical structure identification.

Along with the discovery of artemisinin, the team carried out an acute toxicity test on laboratory rats, as well as histopathologic examinations on main organs, such as heart, liver, spleen, lung, kidney, and brain of rats, cats and other animals; in addition, three scientific researchers also participated in the drug trial of artemisinin.

Animal toxicity tests and human drug trial showed that artemisinin had no obvious impact on other visceral organs except for slight or transient impact on a few animals and people, thus fully indicating the white needle crystals only had a slight toxic and side effect.

Tu Youyou also considered the matter of whether the mass production of artemisinin could be realized. Beijing-grown *Artemisia annua* L. contains lots of impurities, and the artemisinin contained could only be extracted through complex methods with a large amount of ether, rendering it unsuitable for use in mass production. Therefore, the team also extracted artemisinin with the "dilute alcohol extraction method" and "solvent gasoline extraction method", which solved the problem of solvent amount to a great extent.

The extraction of needle crystals was a declaration that the extraction of artemisinin and even the turning of artemisinin crystal into drug would no longer only be "a matter of scientific research". For institutes around China, it was no longer an unattainable hope to produce artemisinin-based drugs, but practicable work that was within reach.

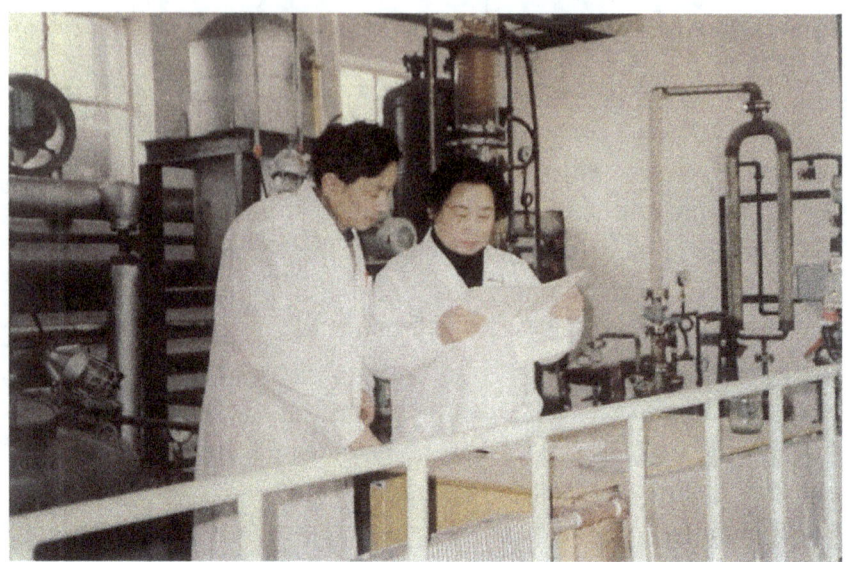

Breathtaking Clinical Trials

In August 1973, the Academy of Chinese Medical Sciences commissioned a foreign pharmaceutical factory to produce the first batch of artemisinin tablets. A medical team formed by Li Chuanjie, Liu Jufu and other researchers was sent to Hainan Changjiang Malaria Area again to carry out clinical verification. Unexpectedly, the tablets only took effect on three of the five clinical patients, and the efficacy was far inferior to previous experimental result.

Facing such a result, the team was not discouraged, but began looking for defects in the tablets. After a short period of testing, they found the cause: there was nothing wrong with artemisinin, it was the tablets that caused the problem. The method of making artemisinin into tablets was problematic, thus affecting disintegration. "Disintegration" refers to the time for a drug to pass through a specific screen after completely dissolving in a specific environment, such as water, intestinal juice or gastric juice. The disintegration time of the artemisinin tablets was too long, so artemisinin was discharged with residual tablets before absorption. Under such circumstances, artemisinin could not be optimally absorbed by the human body.

It was the Cultural Revolution Period, and it was hard to produce artemisinin tablets due to the closure of the drug manufacturing room of the Institute of Chinese Materia Medica. The research team decided to produce capsules, which, compared with tablets, could be made using a simpler process, and also allow the active ingredient to be more easily released for human body absorption.

Later on, due to time urgency, the capsules, which had not yet undergone the disintegration test, were taken to Hainan Changjiang Malaria Area for clinical curative effect observation by Zhang Guozheng, Deputy Director of the Institute of Chinese Material Medica, China Academy of Chinese Medical Sciences. Researchers offered three clinical patients capsules with the dose of 3–3.5 g, and all were cured. In addition, plasmodia were, on average, eliminated in 18.5 h, and the fever subsidence time was 30 h, showing an obvious effect. The researchers, reading the trial report, were visibly relieved.

As such, the initial clinical trial of artemisinin-based medicine was successfully completed. In the meantime, various clinical trials on artemisinin were also being carried out around China. By 1978, 529 cases of clinical trials had been completed in China, all of which achieved good results.

A Large Stage in China

In October 1973, researchers of the Institute of Chinese Materia Medica returned to Beijing and made a report to the "523" Office. On November 2, the office wrote a letter to the Academy of Chinese Medical Sciences, and called for an "Antimalarial Drugs (Including Synthetic Drugs) Research Meeting" to discuss the issue of "developing novel drugs through combination of Chinese traditional and Western medicine". The instruction was clear: "artemisinin is a critical drug, please organize and prepare the relevant materials for discussion". Tu Youyou made a comprehensive report again at the meeting.

In February 1974, the Academy of Chinese Medical Sciences chaired the "Artemisinin Thematic Research Symposium" which disclosed, for the first time, the relevant findings of artemisinin research laboratories under the institute, allowed participants to tour the premises and also receive a detailed introduction. Later, institutes from Sichuan Province, Guangxi Province, and Guangdong Province also participated in the research. According to statistics, more than 40 units participated in the antimalarial research and carried out 6,555 clinical trials.

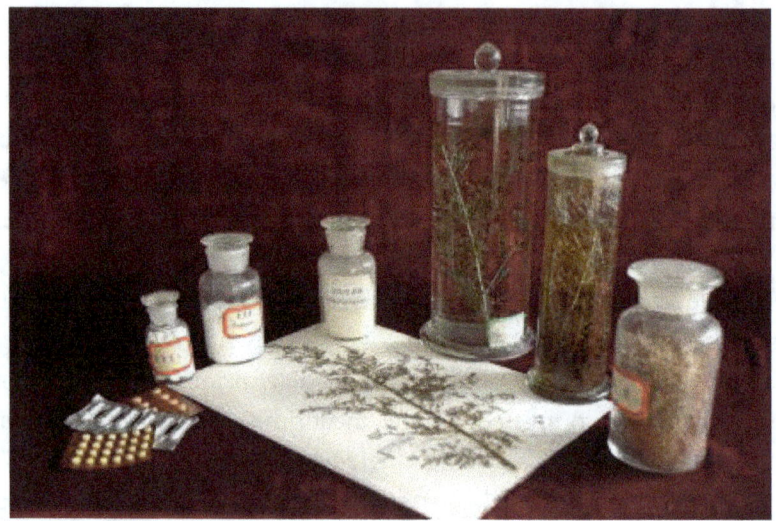

From right to left: *Artemisia annua* L. specimen, artemisinin, and artemisinin-based medicine.

On the large antimalarial stage in China, artemisinin-based medicine quickly became a shining star.

Unique Artemisinin

Artemisinin, a kind of white needle crystal with a melting point of 156–157°C, was confirmed through chemical reaction and other various tests to contain no nitrogen; with a formula of $C_{15}H_{22}O_5$ and a molecular weight of 282, it is a typical organic compound.

At a conspicuous position in Tu's laboratory, there is a 3D model of the structure of artemisinin, it is clearly a proud achievement, and object of her lifelong research.

As a matter of fact, it took some time to determine the structure of artemisinin.

After successful extraction of artemisinin at lower temperature, Tu's team wanted to know the inner structure of artemisinin and how it could cure malaria.

Kekule and the Benzene Ring

Tu thought of the story of the German chemist Kekule, who had discovered the ring formula of benzene in the mid-19th century with his unremitting efforts. Before his discovery, people were confused about how benzene could maintain a stable chemical property even though its carbon atoms are in a highly unsaturated state. Kekule solved the problem by drawing a hexagonal ring on paper, which is the benzene ring that we all now know.

It is an interesting story, for Kekule discovered the benzene ring not by studying textbooks or classics, but from a dream. It was a snowy day around 1864–1865, Kekule had dozed off beside the fireplace whilst reading a complicated research report.

A few seconds later, a dizzy Kekule found himself in darkness without fireplace, carpet, rocking chair, window and house. There was a snake flying slowly in the vast empty space, just like the embodiment of a constellation. Frightened, Kekule could not move; rooted to the spot, he found himself watching the eyes of that snake. All of a sudden, the snake opened its eyes wide, put its tongue out and bit its tail, forming an irregular ring in the air.

Kekule suddenly woke up and looked around, everything appeared normal. He seemed to see the letters representing the elements in benzene twist and turn around the warm flames of the fire. Suddenly, he exclaimed in delight and hastily put pen to paper, what he drew was the first representation of the "benzene ring" in the world.

New Drug without Nitrogen

Motivated by the story, Tu Youyou also believed it was not important where inspiration came from, but that the most important thing was to explore all kinds of possibilities, both in reality and the imaginary like Kekule, and to grasp the transient inspiration when it strikes. Along this line of thought, she focused her attention on test reports, and seemingly, the data appeared to become much clearer.

On November 8, 1972, the research team officially began their research on the chemical structure of artemisinin. After conducting the conventional elemental analysis, Tu Youyou and her colleagues were surprised to find that artemisinin, compared with chinoline-based antimalarial drugs, contained no nitrogen atoms, but only consisted of the elements: carbon, hydrogen and oxygen. What they found shocked everyone, for in those years, people believed the key antimalarial factor was nitrogen. They were quite excited at such a discovery, and believed they would soon reveal a new compound, which would be a great discovery worthy of record in the annals of history.

With greater research, its appearance was gradually revealed: Artemisinin, a kind of white needle crystal with a melting point of 156–157°C, was confirmed through chemical reaction and other various tests to be a typical organic compound. It contained no nitrogen, had a formula of $C_{15}H_{22}O_5$ and a molecular weight of 282. Under the guidance and analysis of Professor Lin Qishou, its "identity" was also determined: it was an antimalarial drug with a new structure belonging to sesquiterpene lactone.

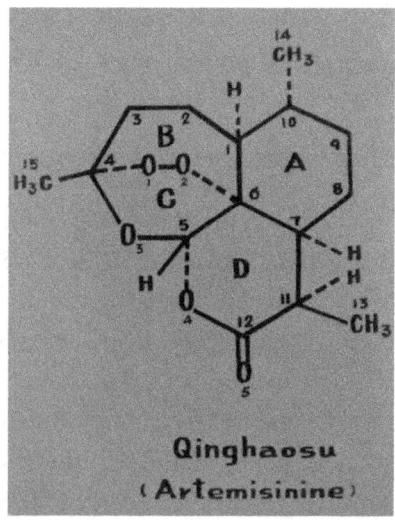

Plane structure of artemisinin, a sesquiterpene lactone.

Terpenoids

Sesquiterpene lactone? What specialties do terpenoids have?

Terpenoids are a large and diverse class of naturally occurring organic chemicals with wide biological activities. At the same time, they are found in physiologically active compounds of Chinese herbs that are widespread in the natural world. With a simple chemical structure set up with five carbon atoms as the "skeleton", they are usually the polymers or derivatives of isoprene (C_5H_8). In general, the terpenoids can be classified according to the number of isoprene units, such as Monoterpenoids, Sesquiterpenoids and Diterpenoids. While "lactones" refer to the cyclic esters with the removal of one water molecule from hydroxyl (-OH) carboxyl (-COOH). Sesquiterpene lactones contained in *Artemisia annua* L. have the functions of cardiac strengthening, tumor prevention, desinsectization and analgesia, amongst others. Therefore, artemisinin naturally belongs to one kind of sesquiterpene lactones.

Three-Dimensional Structure

"In addition to the plane structure, we shall determine its three-dimensional structure." In 1973, the Institute of Chinese Materia Medica started preparing the research scheme to determine the three-dimensional structure of artemisinin. In 1974, Tu Youyou took the relevant materials to the Shanghai Institute of Organic Chemistry, to visit Professor Liu Zhujin who possessed rich research experience on sesquiterpenes. The Institute of Chinese Materia Medica divided the research responsibilities as follows: Ni Muyun was to leverage on the strengths of the Shanghai Institute of Organic Chemistry to carry out further research; meanwhile, Tu Youyou was to take charge of cooperation with the Institute of Biophysics, Chinese Academy of Sciences in Beijing, to cultivate crystals required by research and provide the relevant data.

In late 1974, the China Academy of Chinese Medical Sciences, in collaboration with the Institute of Biophysics, Chinese Academy of Sciences, conducted identification on the structure of artemisinin with the X-ray diffraction method. X-ray diffraction refers to the method of identifying the trajectory of X-ray reflected by carbon, hydrogen, and oxygen atoms in crystals. The reflection trajectory is determined by the nature of atoms. Experimentalists can judge and analyze different atoms in crystals through the reflection trajectory of X-ray; thus the atomic structure of each crystal can be accurately determined.

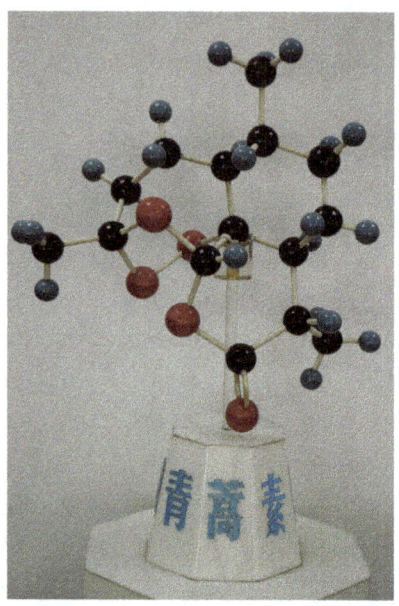

Three-dimensional structure of artemisinin.

On November 30, 1975, basic X-ray diffraction work was smoothly completed, and the chemical structure of artemisinin was preliminarily determined. In order to ensure the accuracy of the chemical structure of artemisinin, the researchers further reviewed X-ray diffraction data after communicating with Professor Liang Xiaotian, and they finally determined the structure of artemisinin.

On January 26, 1976, Tu Youyou and Li Pengfei from the Institute of Biophysics took a flight to the Shanghai Institute of Organic Chemistry to report the identification status of artemisinin's structure. On the next day, Li Pengfei made a report on how the chemical structure of artemisinin was determined with the X-ray diffraction method. Zhou Weishan, Wu Yulin, Wu Zhaohua and other experts participated in the meeting, detailed analysis and thorough discussion ensued. After reaching a consensus, the China Academy of Chinese Medical Sciences reported the relevant achievements of the meeting to the Party Committee of the Ministry of Health of the People's Republic of China. At that moment, the three-dimensional structure of artemisinin was finally confirmed. In 1976, the Academy of Chinese Medical Sciences submitted Document No. 17 *Issue on Publishing Information about Artemisinin Structure Determination* to the leaders of Ministry of Health to ask for instructions on whether the relevant research results could be published.

Finally, with the approval of the Ministry of Health, *A New-Type Sesquiterpene — Artemisinin* was published in the *Chinese Science Bulletin* in March 1977; soon afterwards, the article attracted attention from the scientific community at home and abroad, and artemisinin was then listed in the US-based registry *Chemical Abstracts*.

> *Considering the confidentiality requirements and the nature of the era, the authorship of the article was attributed to "Artemisinin Structure Research Cooperative Team". Artemisinin thus made its first appearance to the rest of the world, but its main discoverer and countless participants in the discovery process remained unknown to the world for many years afterwards.*

Rectification of the Name of *Artemisia annua* L.

With several different botanical varieties on the domestic market all being sold as Artemisia annua L., Tu's team, after discovering artemisinin, painstakingly distinguished all the varieties of Artemisia annua L., and eventually isolated six that could be considered for use.

In order to better develop artemisinin, Tu Youyou carried out research on *Artemisia annua* L., the medical herb containing artemisinin. She surveyed *Artemisia annua* L. at medicine markets in different regions of China and collected ten batches of *Artemisia annua* L. materials for experimental research. The process included pharmacological research on the antipyretic, anti-inflammatory, analgesic and anti-bacteria functions of *Artemisia annua* L., and also research on cultivation and breeding of *Artemisia annua* L. Tu's laboratory also tried improving *Artemisia annua* L. through space mutation breeding.

What is *Artemisia annua* L.?

Back during 1934–1937, Tu's college teacher Zhao Yuhuang had already questioned the varieties of *Artemisia annua* L. growing in Beijing.

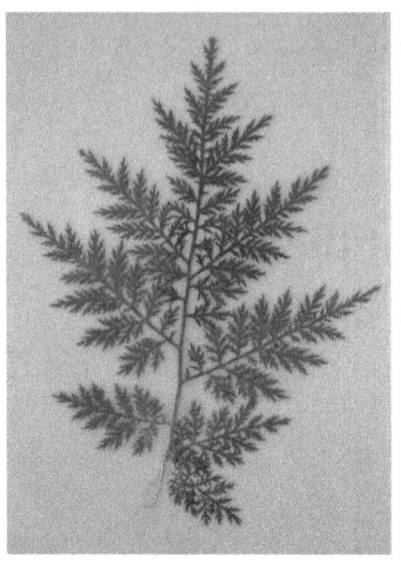

A Japanese scholar once pointed out in a report that "... *Artemisia annua* L. listed in *Compendium of Materia Medica* is similar to common seseli". Through long-term research, he found that what was used for medicine in Beijing was "*Artemisia annua · Artemisia hedinii*" different from the *Artemisia annua* included in the *Compendium of Materia Medica*. Zhao's unremitting efforts corrected the error of classifying *Artemisia apiacea* hence as *Artemisia annua* L. in the *Chinese Pharmacopoeia* (ed. 1963, 1977). Today, scholars including Chen Chongming have verified that *Artemisia apiacea* hance should be common seseli, and should not be classified within the scope of *Artemisia annua* L. The efforts taken by Zhao Yuhuang were finally affirmed.

Six Varieties of *Artemisia annua* L.

With several different botanical varieties on the domestic market all being sold as *Artemisia annua* L., Tu's team, after discovering artemisinin, painstakingly distinguished all the varieties of *Artemisia annua* L, and eventually isolated six that could be considered for use.

Artemisia annua L.

Being popular among the masses, it has many interesting and lovely names in Chinese, including Chouhao, Xianghao, Caohao, Qinghao, Chouqinghao, Xiangqinghao, Xiyehao, and Caohaozi. As a kind of therophyte herb, it mainly grows in fields, on hillsides, and along the sides of roads and rivers. Throughout China, it is possible to find courtyards full of *Artemisia annua* L. emanating a sweet fragrance.

Common seseli

Unlike its name, it is not common. Fine and smooth in appearance, it prefers growing in sandy ground and alongside rivers and seas, especially in Northeast China, South China and Southwest China.

Artemisia scoparia

This is a kind of therophyte to perennial herb with indomitable vitality that vertically sinks its firm spindle- and cone-shaped roots into the ground. As a representative of toughness, *Artemisia scoparia* prefers harsh environments, such as by the side of ditches and hills, gravelly ground and saline-alkali soil.

Artemisia capillaries

This is a perennial herb. As "the small centipede" in the family of *Artemisia annua* L., it has a unique conical root stalk and often grows obliquely. It prefers beaches and the coast, as well as sandy ground by the riversides in China's eastern and southern coastal provinces, a few prefer living on hillsides in offshore regions.

Artemisia japonica

This is the "Optimus Prime" in the family of *Artemisia annua* L., and a kind of perennial herb with the height of 50–150 cm. The branches at the upper portion of the plant always spread like petals.

Artemisia eriopoda

Being different from *Artemisia japonica*, *Artemisia eriopoda*, as the "little golden bean" in the family of *Artemisia annua* L., is only 30–70 cm high, but stands tall upright. It prefers living in clusters, but also occasionally grows separately. There are dense fuzzy hairs covering the roots.

The Artemisia annua L. used for extracting artemisinin had been accidentally found by the side of a road in the suburbs of Beijing by Tu Youyou. It was confirmed to be the authentic Artemisia annua L. after a cautious identification process. Tu once said, "Perhaps, this is the key to success." That herb found by Tu was soon processed into extract in a test tube; through a complex process, artemisinin was successfully extracted.

Each Showing Its Special Prowess

The special structure and outstanding therapeutic effect of artemisinin prompted domestic and overseas researchers to find out more about its chemical components. So far, more than 170 compounds have been isolated and various types of antimalarial drugs developed, each of which shows its special prowess on the antimalarial battlefield.

Artemisinin

In the pharmaceutical field, the determination of artemisinin's chemical structure not only gave humankind knowledge of a new compound but also the first highly effective antimalarial drug.

In 1979, artemisinin won the State Award for Inventions.

In 1986, artemisinin was awarded China's first A-Class *New Drug Certificate* [(1986) No. X-01] after implementation of provisions for new drug approval; it became the only innovative drug originating from China that is recognized by the international community; it was praised as "a model for new drug development from traditional Chinese medicine".

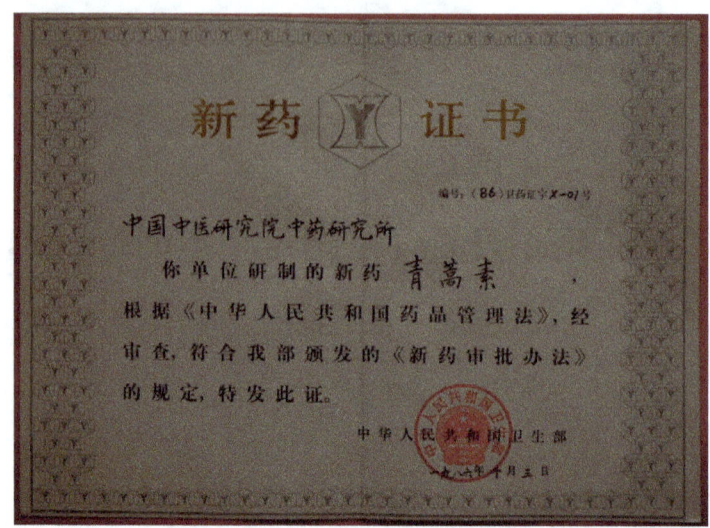

New drug certificate of artemisinin.

In 1981, the "Artemisinin and its Derivatives" conference hosted by the UNDP and SWG-Chemal of the WHO (World Health Organization) was held in Beijing. At this important meeting, the participating representatives critically evaluated and attributed high value to artemisinin.

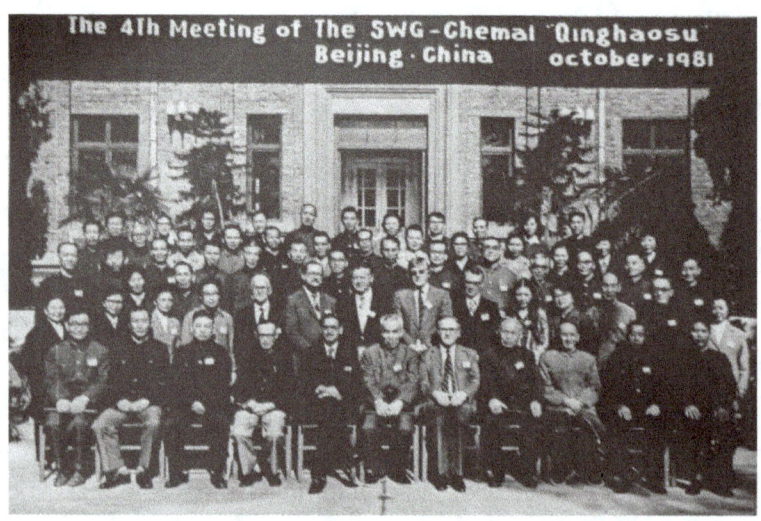

The "Artemisinin and its Derivatives" conference hosted by SWG-Chemal was held in Beijing.

Dihydroartemisinin

The special structure and outstanding therapeutic effect of artemisinin prompted domestic and overseas researchers to find out more about its chemical components. So far, more than 170 compounds have been isolated and various types of antimalarial drugs developed, each of which shows its special prowess on the antimalarial battlefield.

In 1973, whilst doing further research on artemisinin and its derivatives at the Institute of Chinese Materia Medica, Tu and her team discovered, for the first time, a derivative of artemisinin — dihydroartemisinin, with the molecular formula of $C_{15}H_{24}O_5$, and relative molecular mass of 284.

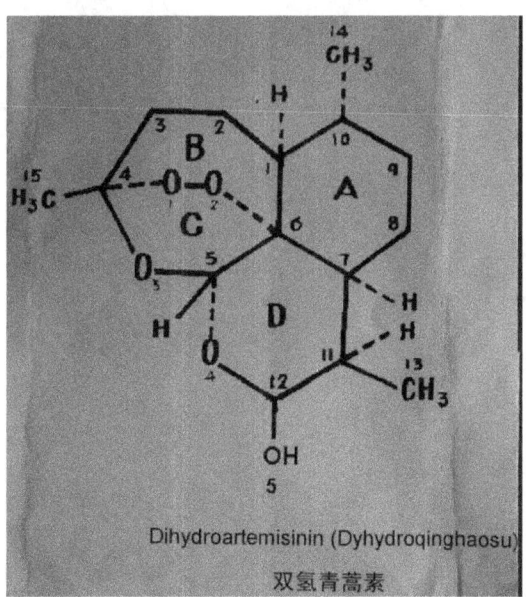

Structure of dihydroartemisinin.

Later, in the continuing study on artemisinin and its derivatives, they synthesized three ether and ten ester derivatives on the basis of dihydroartemisinin. In this process, Tu and her colleagues proved that peroxide forms the main antimalarial active groups in the structure of artemisinin through a large number of rodent malaria efficacy detections. As long as the peroxide active groups were preserved, their special derivatives could greatly improve the efficacy of artemisinin.

Therefore, at the national collaboration meeting held in 1975, dihydroartemisinin became a "sweet pastry". With the relationship between structure and efficacy determined by Tu's team, dihydroartemisinin had the potential to become a new antimalarial drug. In the following seven years, dihydroartemisinin, with continual research, improvement and perfection, also became another new drug attaining "Class A" status and independent patent rights; it was also one of the winners of the "1992 National Awards for Top Ten Scientific Achievements".

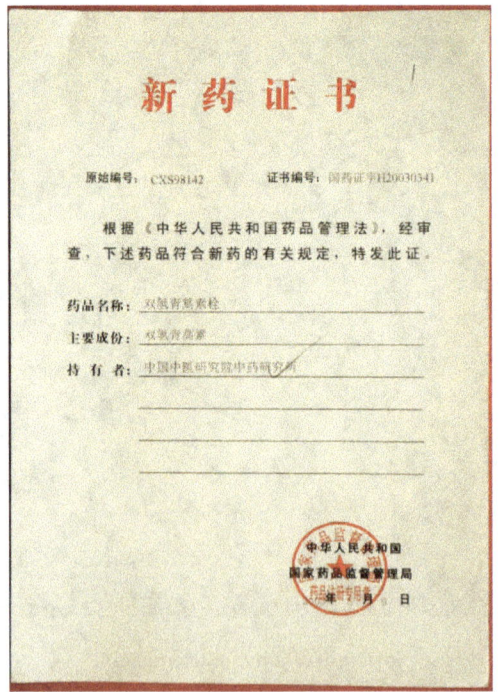

New drug certificate of dihydroartemisinin suppositories.

In addition to Tu's team that developed dihydroartemisinin, many other drug research institutions also conducted research on artemisinin-based drugs and successfully developed many effective drugs.

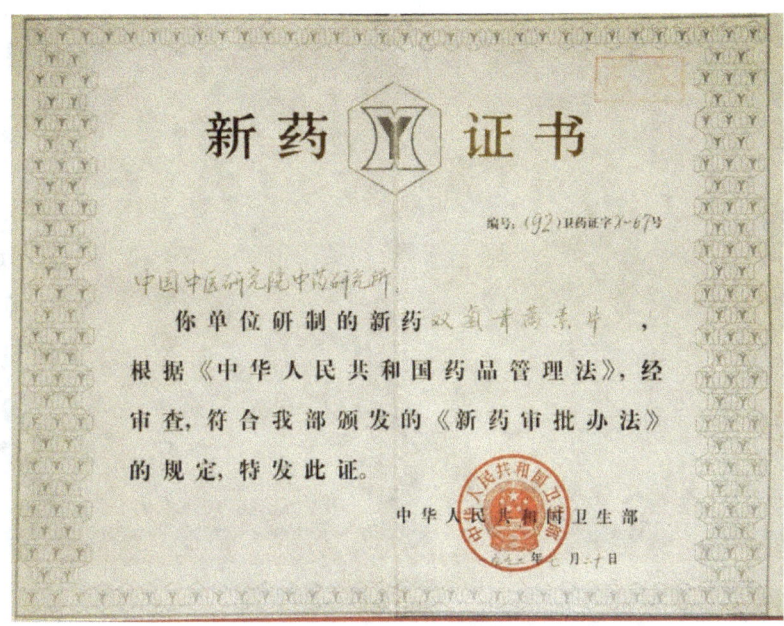

New drug certificate of dihydroartemisinin tablets.

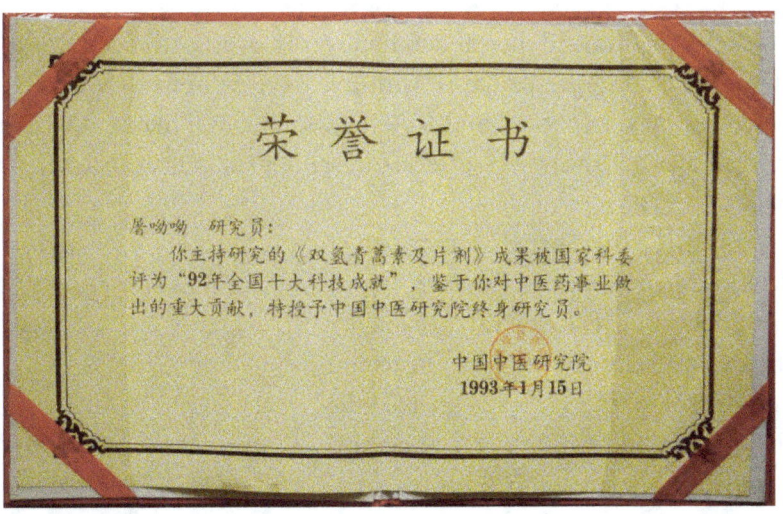

Tu Youyou was a winner of the "1992 National Awards for Top Ten Scientific Achievements"; she was hired as a lifelong researcher by the Academy of Chinese Medical Sciences.

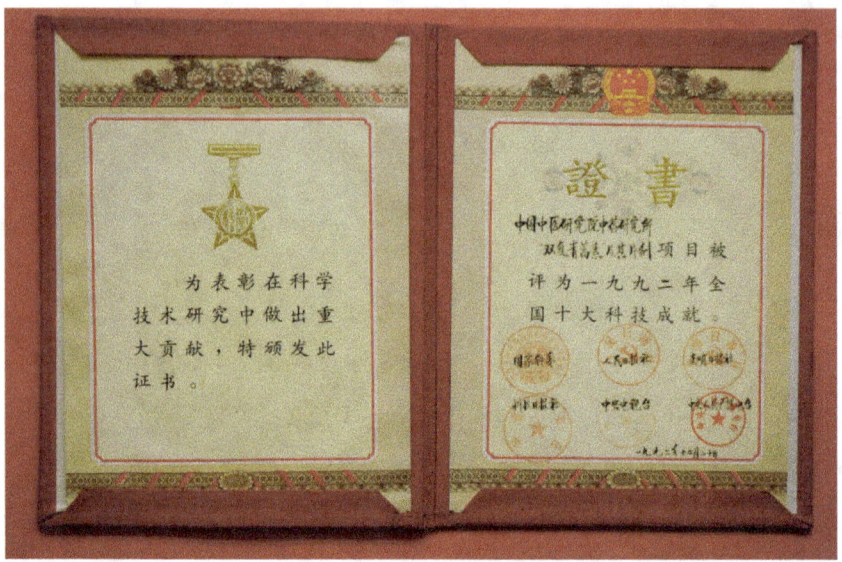

The project of dihydroartemisinin and its tablets was a winner in the "1992 National Awards for Top Ten Scientific Achievements".

The Popular Artemether

In late 1975, Tu and her team finally discovered the structure of artemisinin: a unique structure with five oxygen atoms in a molecule connected by ketal, acetal and lactone, which is the material basis for curing malaria. However, it suffers from a poor solubility during clinical trials.

In 1976, the Shanghai Institute of Materia Medica started looking for a new artemisinin compound with higher efficacy and solubility through structural transformation. In 1977, they selected the ether compound "SM 224" — "Artemether" among tens of other compounds.

Atomic structure of Artemether.

Artemether, with stable chemical properties, is suitable to be taken as oily injection. In 1977, clinical trials of Artemether were started. The first clinical trial on 17 patients was conducted in Hainan Province, and achieved excellent effects. In the subsequent three years, Artemether successfully cured 1,088 malaria patients from areas in Hainan, Yunnan, Guangxi, Henan, Hubei and other provinces, and realized the curative rate of 100% in treating patients with falciparum malaria.

In clinical application, Artemether is quite popular among patients and medical staff. In addition to the stable curative effect to chloroquine-resistant falciparum malaria, it rarely causes soreness post-injection.

Efficient Artesunate

In 1977, in Guangxi Province, rich in *Artemisia annua* L. resources, Guangxi Guilin Pharmaceutical Factory also began research on artemisinin derivatives. Following the guidelines by the Shanghai Institute of Materia Medica, Guilin Pharmaceutical Factory, Guangxi Medical University and Guangxi Institute of Parasitic Diseases jointly synthesized more than ten artemisinin derivatives, of which No. 804 had the most outstanding efficacy.

In Guangxi Province, an Artemisinin Derivatives Research Cooperative Team was established to carry out the elemental analysis, as well as chemical structure determination with infrared spectroscopy, mass-spectrography and nuclear magnetic resonance method; it also conducted an X-ray diffraction research with the assistance of the Institute of Biophysics, Chinese Academy of Sciences. Finally, the chemical structure

Atomic structure of Artesunate.

of Derivative No. 804 was revealed. In October 1978, clinical trials on Derivative No. 804 were started. In the process of curing 24 patients (9 with falciparum malaria and 15 with tertian malaria), only 300 mg of 804-sodium powder injection was used. Later, its highly efficient, quick-acting and low-toxicity features were widely spread throughout China.

In 1979, Derivative No. 804 was officially named "Artesunate" and published in the *Chinese Pharmaceutical Bulletin* (X-01); at present, it is used as an important drug for treating cerebral malaria all around the world.

Coartem

In the 1980s, the research on artemisinin carried out by China took the lead amongst international research on antimalarial drugs. Among the research institutions which contributed most is the Institute of Microbiology and Epidemiology, Academy of Military Medical Sciences. Since 1951, many other institutions, from Hainan to Shanghai, have been engaging in the development of antimalarial drugs.

In 1990, the Institute of Microbiology and Epidemiology, Academy of Military Medical Sciences, became the first institution to successfully develop the Artemether-Benflumetol compound prescription. The compound drug Benflumetol takes effect slowly, but allows for the complementary advantages assorted with Artemether and other fast acting drugs to be realized, thus creating an obvious catalytic effect. Artemether-Benflumetol was approved as a new drug with "Class C" status and granted with a New Drug Certificate and Production Approval Document in April 1992 after complex research and testing. It is also the first compound artemisinin-based drug developed in China.

In June 2009, the development team of "Artemether-Benflumetol" won the "European Inventor Award" — the highest award for inventions in Europe in 2009.

> *Scientific researchers around China gradually participated in the research, and more and more artemisinin-based drugs were developed, enlarging the family of artemisinin-based drugs ...*

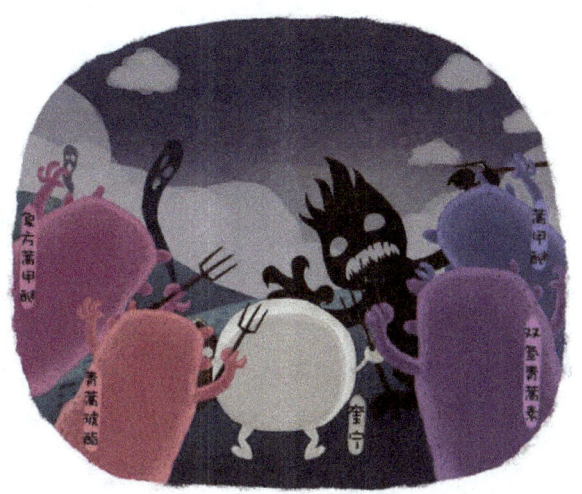

Family of artemisinin-based drugs (drawn by Zhang Linhao).

Introduction into Africa

―•―‡◊‡―•―

When she was dying, the casually obtained drug "COTECXIN" saved her life. More miraculously, her unborn fetus was also saved. She can never forget the moment that she was able to call out to her little baby "COTECXIN". She said in an interview, "I named my baby 'COTECXIN' not just because I want to show gratitude, but also because I hope he will inherit the strength of COTECXIN, to develop Kenya and protect it from being attacked by malaria forever."

The development of artemisinin and artemisinin-based drugs began to draw extensive attention from the international community, but the path for artemisinin to go international from China was not a smooth one.

Artemisia annua L. Farming

Before the discovery of artemisinin, *Artemisia annua* L. was seldom used as medicine, when used, it was mainly *Artemisia annua* L. that had grown in the wild. However, once artemisinin was discovered, there was a surge in demand for *Artemisia annua* L.

During the country-wide investigation for artemisinin resources carried out in the 1970s, the wild ones growing in clusters in Youyang, Sichuan Province were selected as raw materials for artemisinin scientific research and clinical trials owing to their large numbers, high quality, and high artemisinin content.

The Artemisinin Steering Committee, founded in 1978, realized the value of *Artemisia annua* L. in Youyang, and began to protect and develop this local resource. The surge in demand for artemisinin drove the development of *Artemisia annua* L. farming; in the eyes of local farmers, *Artemisia annua* L. gradually became "a hen laying golden eggs". More and more farmers enthusiastically planted *Artemisia annua* L., thus creating supply for establishing an industry. In the meantime, the process of marketization in China also began, which became the first step in preparations for the internationalization of artemisinin.

Establishment of Pharmaceutical Factories

Although the source of *Artemisia annua* L. was guaranteed, the backwardness of existing technology and equipment made it difficult to widely utilize those raw materials. For this reason, local governments in China started establishing pharmaceutical factories, which then gradually turned the accumulated *Artemisia annua* L. into antimalarial drugs.

In 1986, the Institute of Chinese Materia Medica, after gaining the New Drug Certificate for artemisinin, established a new production base in Jishou, Hunan Province taking advantage of the high quality of *Artemisia annua* L. locally to rapidly manufacture artemisinin in large quantities. Soon afterwards, the artemisinin refinery project — Wuling Mountain Pharmaceutical Factory was established and put into service in Youyang, hometown of excellent *Artemisia annua* L. Considering the poverty in Youyang, the Artemisinin Steering Committee specially allocated funds and asked the Shandong Academy of Chinese Medicine to participate in the project, to resolve any issues with regard to production equipment and techniques. In September 1987, Wuling Mountain Pharmaceutical Factory finally succeeded in producing certified artemisinin-based drugs, representing the completion and operation of the first ton-level artemisinin factory in China.

Since then, various kinds of new artemisinin-based antimalarial drugs have been developed, such as Artemether oily injection, Artesunate water injection, Dihydroartemisinin tablets and Artemether-Benflumetol compound. From 1985 when the regulations for new drug evaluation was implemented in China to 1995, the government approved a total of 14 new Class A drugs, seven of which were artemisinin-based new antimalarial drugs.

Story of DDT

At that time, the WHO paid more attention to the influence of artemisinin-based drugs on the human body and ecological balance, notwithstanding their therapeutic effects and side effects. In the approval process of each new drug, WHO researchers always had one concern at the back of their minds: DDT.

DDT is a kind of pesticide which played a large role in preventing agricultural pests and reducing the mosquito- and fly-borne diseases including malaria and typhoid fever in the first half of the 20th century. DDT's insecticidal properties were discovered by the Swiss scientist Paul Hermann Müller, who was awarded the 1948 Nobel Prize in Physiology and Medicine for his efforts.

Silent Spring, a book written by Rachel Carson and published in 1962, begins in a beautiful fictional city. One day, the city becomes enshrouded in a strange silence, and all the beauty in it begins to vanish. The "silence" was attributed to DDT being widely used in farms across the country. Based on Carson's research on DDT usage in USA farms, the book was seen as an attack on DDT and naturally drew strong opposition from farmers, pesticide manufacturers and others with vested interests who sought to downplay the veracity of the book. Carson and her supporters were greatly depressed that people did not realize the detrimental effects of pesticides. It was not until President John F. Kennedy read the book and ordered an investigation into all the pesticides mentioned that the tide began to turn. People realized DDT would accumulate in bodies of animals, enter into the food chain, thus causing reproductive system disorders and extinction of birds. In fact, the national bird of the United States, the bald eagle, became extinct due to DDT.

The Humble New Drug

Given the lesson from DDT, the WHO was understandably more cautious in reviewing and endorsing new drugs. In March 1982, SWG-CHEMAL of the WHO decided on Artesunate as the preferential development project, and sent specialists to China to check on the production processes of Chinese factories and plants. Although full preparations were made, Kunming Pharmaceutical Factory, Guilin No. 1 and 2 Pharmaceutical Factory, and even Shanghai Sine Pharma with the best conditions, failed to pass the test of Good Manufacturing Practice (GMP).

In 1990, the development of the drug, Coartem, changed everything. Novartis, one of the world's top three pharmaceutical enterprises, ventured into China in that year, and Chinese pharmaceutical companies made full preparations and introduced all artemisinin-based antimalarial drugs to Novartis in detail, including various high-profile antimalarial drugs in China. However, due to expiry of the patent protection duration for many of them, there was a concern by Novartis that there would be patent disputes in foreign countries, thus all the drugs were all rejected. Eventually, it was Coartem, despite its relatively brief introduction in comparison to the other more high-profile drugs, that was finally selected by Novartis. But it had not obtained the New Drug Certificate at the time of Novartis' selection.

On September 12, 1994, Novartis signed a 20-year *Cooperation Agreement* with China, and then formally signed the *Patent Licensing Agreement* on September 20, 2004. By 1999, Coartem had gained the patents for invention in 49 countries and regions in the world, passed the drug registration in 84 countries and regions; and in the same year, it was included in the WHO's "Essential Drugs List". It became the first artemisinin-based combination drug passing the quality review of WHO and UNICEF around the world.

Countries with malaria outbreaks use Coartem, with a clinical curative rate of 97%, as the first-line drug. It is an internationally accepted drug with the best efficacy in treating drug-resistant malaria, and also one of only three patented drugs that have been listed in the WHO's "Essential Drugs List" for the past 25 years.

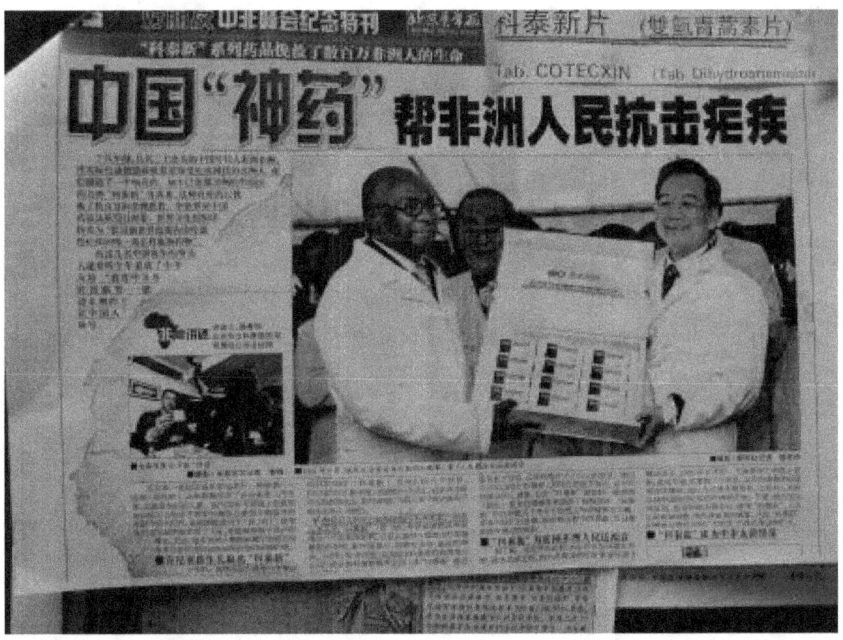

"Chinese Miracle Drug Helps Africa Fight Malaria"

Magical COTECXIN

On the vast African continent, Dihydroartemisinin has created its own miracle. "COTECXIN", a kind of dihydroartemisinin drug developed by Beijing Holley-Cotec Pharmaceuticals Co., Ltd., was introduced into Kenya in October 1993. Being different from Coartem, dihydroartemisinin was distributed via private purchasing, and was promoted through usage by common people. From October 1993 to 1999, "COTECXIN" became "an antimalarial legend" in Kenya. At present, 80% of Kenyans know "COTECXIN", even taxi drivers and ordinary farmers will give a thumbs up when it is mentioned.

To Kenyans, the feeling they have toward "COTECXIN" is beyond gratitude. There was a report in 2001 of a baby born in an impoverished mountainous area in Kenya's capital Nairobi; his parents who had been cured from malaria did not agonise over naming him, instead, at first sight of her child, his mother called out, "COTECXIN...COTECXIN...".

"COTECXIN" is the commercial name of the antimalarial drug dihydroartemisinin.

In those years, malaria was cruelly attacking weak pregnant women in Kenya and the rest of the African continent. Many fetuses died in utero. The mother mentioned above was one of the pregnant women who suffered greatly from malaria; however, "COTECXIN" saved her life. More miraculously, her unborn fetus was also saved. She can never forget the moment that she was able to call out to her little baby "COTECXIN". She said in an interview, "I named my baby 'COTECXIN' not just because I want to show gratitude, but also because I hope he will inherit the strength of COTECXIN, to develop Kenya and protect it from being attacked by malaria forever."

> *By the start of the 21st century, artemisinin-based drugs had become widely adopted in the fight against malaria; artemisinin had saved countless lives and prevented the fragmentation of countless families. Still, no one knew who had first discovered it.*

Looking for the Discoverer

Due to historical reasons, the papers and reports published in that era attached more importance to collective rather than individual contributions; therefore, Tu's efforts had been concealed for a long period of time, which is also one of the reasons that there were disputes afterwards about her actual role.

Censure and Dispute

In June 1996, Tu Youyou received a Letter of Invitation from Qiu Shi Science & Technologies Foundation, which had selected her as one of the ten winners of the "Outstanding Scientific and Technological Achievements Collective Award — Artemisinin Award", and invited her to make a fifteen-minute speech at the award ceremony as a keynote speaker.

Tu Youyou, attaching great importance to this invitation, personally wrote back to accept and actively prepared the speech.

At the event held on August 31, Tu Youyou talked about the development course of artemisinin and dihydroartemisinin in chronological order. Unexpectedly, during her speech, a scientist in the audience stood up and censured, "Was artemisinin discovered by you? Leaders of 523 Office are here..." What he meant was that the method of treating malaria with *Artemisia annua* L. had already been recorded in history, and it was not the discovery of any unit or any individual. All of a sudden, the atmosphere became quite tense...

We cannot know for sure how Tu Youyou felt when she left the venue that day, but undoubtedly, it must have been a terrible blow to her.

Due to historical reasons, the papers and reports published in that era attached more importance to collective rather than individual contributions; therefore, Tu's efforts had been concealed for a long period of time, which is also one of the reasons that there were disputes afterwards about her actual role.

Miller's Search

The excellent performance of artemisinin on the international antimalarial battlefield became obvious, and it caught the attention of Louis H. Miller, an academician at the US National Academy of Sciences and expert engaging in malaria research for over fifty years. More importantly, he has the right of nominating Nobel Prize Winners.

In 2007, Miller went to Shanghai to attend a meeting on malaria and its infection medium with Su Xinzhuan, Senior Scientist at the National Institutes of Health. At the meeting, Miller kept asking, who discovered artemisinin? How was it discovered? But no one could answer him. It was inconceivable to Miller, for he could not believe no one knew who had made such a great discovery.

Xinhua News Agency reported what Su Xinzhuan described in an interview: One day, while chatting over lunch with Su, Miller mentioned that artemisinin was an important discovery and could compete with other discoveries for a prize. Su paused, then suggested, perhaps the Nobel Prize. Miller, after thinking for a short while, agreed. At that moment, Miller determined to seek out and recommend the discoverer of artemisinin to the Nobel Prize Committee.

Who should be credited with the discovery of artemisinin? The answer to this question was not generally known when Miller and Su began to delve into the history of the discovery, for relevant reports and papers in China did not mention the discoverer by name; however, history is history and truth is truth, the historical documents and experimental records could not conceal the reality of the past decades.

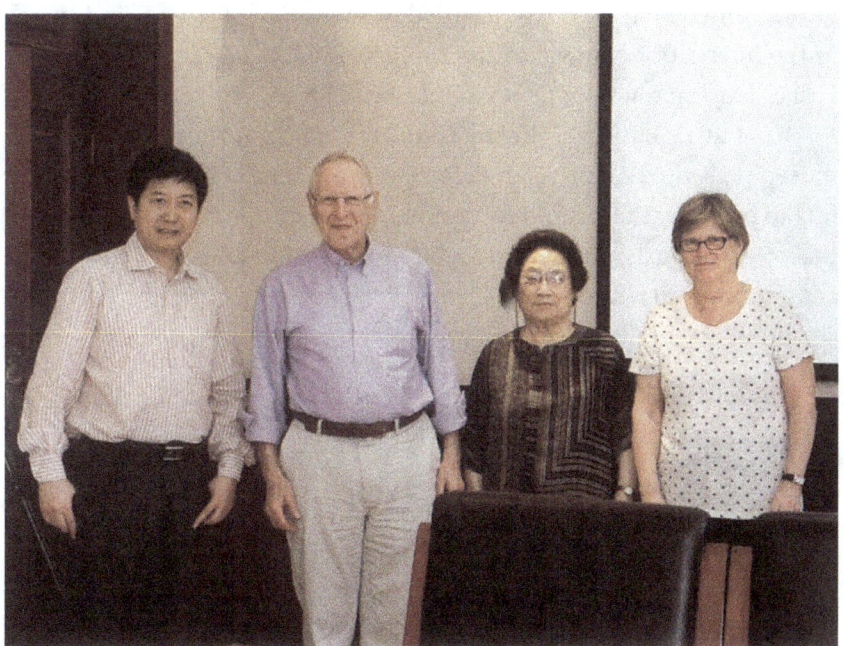

Tu Youyou and Miller (second from left).

When they looked up the historical materials, one name — Tu Youyou — became more and more conspicuous.

Glory to Tu Youyou

An article introducing artemisinin and Tu Youyou's contributions — *Artemisinin: Discovery from the Chinese Herbal Garden* was published by the journal *Cell* in 2011. It introduced, in detail, the establishment of Project 523, the discovery process of artemisinin, and the later clinical trials. At the end, it expressed that whilst the challenges of combating malaria remain daunting, the discovery of artemisinin by Tu Youyou and her many colleagues in the Chinese scientific community offers hope and is a great achievement in the history of modern medicine.

Louis H. Miller and Su Xinzhuan authored this article to nominate Tu Youyou for the 2011 Lasker-DeBakey Clinical Medical Research Award, which, as the most esteemed award in the biomedical sciences in the United States, is also regarded as the "Nobel Prize's Wind Vane" in the international medical community; in fact, a large proportion of Lasker laureates have gone on to receive the Nobel Prize.

The 2011 Lasker-DeBakey Clinical Medical Research Award was indeed presented to Tu Youyou, for the committee believed she was the first to propose artemisinin for serious consideration in Project 523, the first to extract artemisinin with a 100% inhibition ratio, and the first to conduct clinical trials.

In 2011, Tu Youyou flew to the United States and received the honor belonging to her. Louis H. Miller, in every year afterwards, included Tu Youyou on the nomination list submitted to the Nobel Prize Committee.

Winning the Nobel Prize

It also bears her unhesitating decision for personal drug trial, the sorrow and grief she experienced when her little daughter refused to call her "mom" after a long separation, the pain of liver disease induced by ether, the innumerable days and nights spent in the laboratory...

"If I have seen further than others, it is because I have stood upon the shoulders of giants."

Isaac Newton

Behind the Medal

After her winning of the Nobel Prize, various media rushed to report such an honor, but Tu Youyou appeared to be quite calm. She attributed the achievement to the joint efforts of her team, and to forerunners on the antimalarial road.

These forerunners included Ross who discovered the complex life cycle of plasmodia, and Laveran who discovered plasmodia and conducted research on it; like many before and after them, they had used the weapon of science to explore the unknown world.

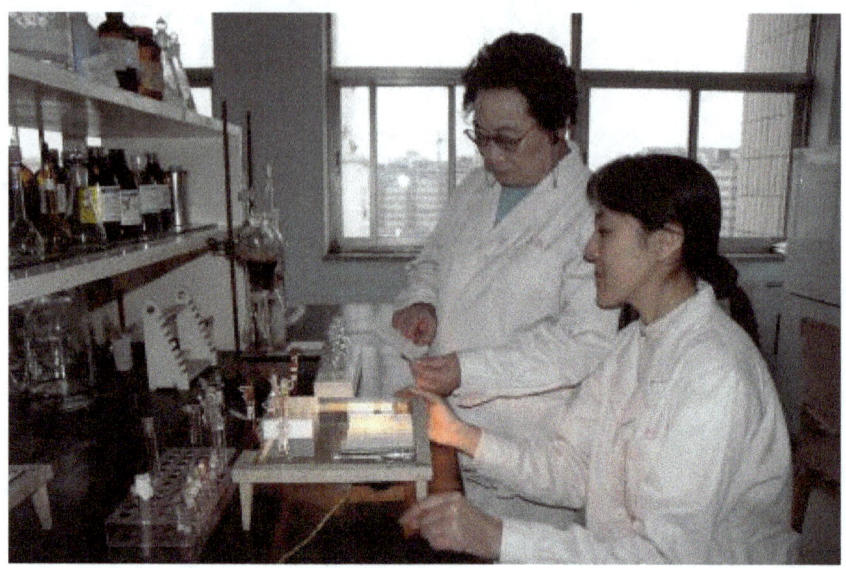

Tu Youyou and her student Yang Lan in the laboratory.

The medal awarded to Tu Youyou seems to bear her childhood dream and record her knowledge-seeking youth in the library of Peking University; it bears her huge stress and strong sense of mission from participating in "Project 523", as well as the excitement when she first successfully extracted artemisinin with ether at low temperature.

Of course, it also bears her unhesitating decision for personal drug trial, the sorrow and grief she experienced when her little daughter refused to call her "mom" after a long separation, the pain of liver disease induced by ether, the innumerable days and nights spent in the laboratory… as well as the smiles and trusting eyes of patients with malaria cured by artemisinin.

Why Her?

But why was Tu Youyou recommended to receive the Nobel Prize?

As mentioned by Goran K. Hansson, Secretary of the Nobel Committee for Physiology or Medicine, the discovery was made by an individual rather than an organization. In such an era where organizations and institutions have great power and have become more important, it is critical to identify the individuals possessing real creativity who have changed the world.

As mentioned, in 2011, the Lasker-DeBakey Clinical Medical Research Award, the most esteemed award in the biomedical sciences, was presented to Tu Youyou, for the Award Committee believed Tu was the first to propose artemisinin in Project 523, the first to extract artemisinin with a 100% inhibition ratio, and the first to conduct clinical trials; each of the three achievements could already enable Tu to win the award. As a matter of fact, when Tu proposed artemisinin to the project team, she became the forerunner in "antimalarial research with *Artemisia annua* L".

> *On the morning of December 4, 2015, citizens in Beijing enjoyed a clear blue sky, a rare sight during the haze season. Tu Youyou carefully checked her luggage, put on a black overcoat, and left for the airport, accompanied by her husband Li Tingzhao. Originally, she had hesitated whether to accept the prize; this eighty-five-year-old lady eventually decided to do so, for as her colleagues had said, it was a great honor to the country. Recalling all important decisions and choices in her research career, serving the country was always a decisive factor for her.*

Epilogue

On December 10, 2015, when Ms. Tu accepted the trophy at the Nobel Prize Award Ceremony, we were proud of her, and also proud to be Chinese.

We wish to show our great respect for Ms. Tu with this book, and to express, as objectively as possible, her growth process as a Chinese female scientist, born in the 1930s, living through the war and turbulent times following the foundation of the New China. We also tried to objectively depict her childhood and school life, as well as those persons and events that had propelled her to engage in scientific research, the choices that had changed her life's path, and sources of strength which had supported her persistence in research.

We thank all members of the team for their contributions to the writing, compiling, revising, printing and marketing of the book; we thank Ms. Tu's students, Mr. Wang Manyuan and Ms. Yang Lan for assistance in providing reference materials; we thank Li Dan of BTV Archives Channel for help in the manuscript; and last but not least, all colleagues who have contributed or assisted in some way toward the publishing of this book.

In the compilation process of the book, a vast amount of material was perused, in the hope of making it as authentic as possible. However, many details have disappeared in history. If there is any erroneous or incomplete content, please do not hesitate to notify us.

Chemical Industry Press
January 2016

www.ingramcontent.com/pod-product-compliance
Lightning Source LLC
Chambersburg PA
CBHW070310230426
43664CB00015B/2707